EXPERIENCING COMPASSION-FOCUSED THERAPY FROM THE INSIDE OUT

SELF-PRACTICE/SELF-REFLECTION GUIDES FOR PSYCHOTHERAPISTS

James Bennett-Levy, Series Editor

This series invites therapists to enhance their effectiveness "from the inside out" using self-practice/self-reflection (SP/SR). Books in the series lead therapists through a structured three-stage process of focusing on a personal or professional issue they want to change, practicing therapeutic techniques on themselves (self-practice), and reflecting on the experience (self-reflection). Research supports the unique benefits of SP/SR for providing insights and skills not readily available through more conventional training procedures. This approach is suitable for therapists at all levels of experience, from trainees to experienced supervisors. Series volumes have a large-size format for ease of use and feature reproducible worksheets and forms that purchasers can download and print. Initial releases cover cognitive-behavioral therapy, schema therapy, and compassion-focused therapy; future titles will cover acceptance and commitment therapy and other evidence-based treatments.

Experiencing CBT from the Inside Out:
A Self-Practice/Self-Reflection Workbook for Therapists
James Bennett-Levy, Richard Thwaites, Beverly Haarhoff, and Helen Perry

Experiencing Schema Therapy from the Inside Out:
A Self-Practice/Self-Reflection Workbook for Therapists
Joan M. Farrell and Ida A. Shaw

Experiencing Compassion-Focused Therapy from the Inside Out:
A Self-Practice/Self-Reflection Workbook for Therapists
Russell L. Kolts, Tobyn Bell, James Bennett-Levy, and Chris Irons

Experiencing Compassion-Focused Therapy from the Inside Out

A Self-Practice/Self-Reflection Workbook for Therapists

Russell L. Kolts
Tobyn Bell
James Bennett-Levy
Chris Irons

Foreword by Paul Gilbert

THE GUILFORD PRESS
New York   London

The authors have checked with sources believed to be reliable in their efforts to provide information
that is complete and generally in accord with the standards of practice that are accepted at the time of
publication. However, in view of the possibility of human error or changes in behavioral, mental health,
or medical sciences, neither the authors, nor the editors and publisher, nor any other party who has been
involved in the preparation or publication of this work warrants that the information contained herein
is in every respect accurate or complete, and they are not responsible for any errors or omissions or the
results obtained from the use of such information. Readers are encouraged to confirm the information
contained in this book with other sources.

Library of Congress Cataloging-in-Publication Data

Names: Kolts, Russell L., editor.
Title: Experiencing compassion-focused therapy from the inside out : a self-practice/self-reflection
    workbook for therapists / Russell L. Kolts and 3 others ; foreword by Paul Gilbert.
Description: New York : The Guilford Press, 2018. | Series: Self-practice/self-reflection guides for
    psychotherapists | Includes bibliographical references and index.
Identifiers: LCCN 2018014465| ISBN 9781462535255 (paperback) | ISBN   9781462535262 (hardcover)
Subjects: LCSH: Emotion-focused therapy. | Compassion. | Cognitive therapy. |
    BISAC: MEDICAL / Psychiatry / General. | SOCIAL SCIENCE / Social Work. |
    PSYCHOLOGY / Psychotherapy / General.
Classification: LCC RC489.F62 E97 2018 | DDC 616.89/1425—dc23
LC record available at *https://lccn.loc.gov/2018014465*

To my parents, John and Mary Kolts—
everything that is good in me comes from you
—R. L. K.

To Alison, Joseph, Dad, Mum,
and all my family for their love and support
—T. B.

To Judy, from whom I have learned so much
about the true nature of compassion
—J. B.-L.

To my grandparents, who each in their own way
showed me what wisdom, strength, and caring commitment are
—C. I.

And to Paul Gilbert, who gave CFT to us all,
and to the community of CFT trainers and practitioners—
may it serve you well

About the Authors

Russell L. Kolts, PhD, is Professor of Psychology at Eastern Washington University. An internationally recognized trainer in compassion-focused therapy (CFT), Dr. Kolts has pioneered the use of CFT in the treatment of problematic anger. He has authored or coauthored numerous scholarly articles and books for both professionals and general readers, including *Buddhist Psychology and CBT: A Practitioner's Guide*. Dr. Kolts has given a TEDx talk entitled "Anger, Compassion, and What It Means to be Strong," and is founding director of the Inland Northwest Compassionate Mind Center in Spokane, Washington.

Tobyn Bell, MSc, is a practitioner of CFT and cognitive-behavioral therapy (CBT) based in Greater Manchester, United Kingdom. He is a CFT trainer for the Compassionate Mind Foundation and a CBT trainer, supervisor, and program lead at the Greater Manchester CBT Training Centre (National Health Service), which is associated with Manchester University. He has published research on mental imagery and compassion and is a registered mental health nurse and trained mindfulness teacher.

James Bennett-Levy, PhD, is Professor of Mental Health and Psychological Well-Being at the University of Sydney, Australia. As a psychotherapy trainer, he has taught in 22 countries, and is one of the most published researchers in the field of therapist training. In particular, he has pioneered and written extensively about self-practice/self-reflection. Dr. Bennett-Levy is coauthor or coeditor of several widely cited books on CBT, including *Experiencing CBT from the Inside Out*. He is Editor of the Guilford series Self-Practice/Self-Reflection Guides for Psychotherapists.

Chris Irons, PhD, DClinPsych, is Co-Director of Balanced Minds, an organization that provides CFT services, training, and resources in London, United Kingdom. He is a board member of the Compassionate Mind Foundation and a Visiting Lecturer at the University of Derby. Since the early 2000s, Dr. Irons has worked with Paul Gilbert and other colleagues on research and clinical developments linked to CFT. He has published numerous articles, book chapters, and books on compassion, attachment, shame, and self-criticism, and regularly provides CFT teaching, training, workshops, and retreats around the world.

Foreword

Psychotherapy is a process by which we use our own minds to try to understand the mind of another and create interactions that will be revelatory, healing, and transformative. In the early days of psychoanalytic psychotherapy, it was recognized that the therapist had to have enough personal insight and awareness to avoid projecting and getting caught up in his or her own defense mechanisms when engaging with the mind of the client. Personal therapy and experience were essential parts of the training (Ellenberger, 1970). This understanding was not a new one: For thousands of years, contemplative traditions recognized that we could not "enlighten" others and help them engage with the inherent suffering of living until we ourselves had traveled that path. For both traditions, insight into oneself was deemed essential.

With the advent of the cognitive and behavioral therapies, interventions became more technological and technique-focused. Behavior modification and exposure, along with cognitive reappraisal, became the focus of interventions, and the mind of the therapist faded into the background. Indeed, in the early days of cognitive-behavioral therapy (CBT), one could become a therapist with very little insight into one's own mind—the therapist might never have personally experienced the therapeutic techniques he or she was applying or advocating because many in CBT didn't emphasize the importance of therapists experiencing the treatments they were delivering. This is a somewhat medical approach, in which one doesn't need to have cancer to treat it, and one doesn't need to have experienced surgery to become a great surgeon. But learning to do psychotherapy is not like learning the technical skills needed by surgeons. It is more like learning to drive and teaching people to drive. In this analogy, your mind is like a car. You may have ridden in a lot of cars, but only by actually driving one do you become good at driving. It is through the *actual experience* of driving that we develop the skill to respond, moment by moment, to the changing conditions of the road. Driving is an extraordinary behavior involving multitasking: one may be changing gears, accelerating or braking, maybe having a conversation, and monitoring other drivers, the conditions of the road, and the direction of travel.

As therapists, we are also required to simultaneously hold many different experiences arising within us. We are detecting and responding automatically to the flow of interactions, making sense of what's happening for our clients, and determining how best to be helpful. Indeed, sometimes we can be so focused on what we think might be the technically correct thing to do that we lose empathic contact with our clients. If you want to become a more skillful driver, you wouldn't just do an online course. You would go on an advanced driving course in which you actually drive over difficult terrain. If you want to become a skilled therapist, technical skills are essential, of course, but having greater insight into your own moment-by-moment process is going to be help you immensely. It raises the issue of declarative versus procedural knowledge, which in many ways is a focus for this book.

This approach of psychotherapy "from the inside out" is a key passion of one of the authors (James Bennett-Levy), who has articulated why technical skill should be matched by learning through self-practice and self-reflection in a way that is central to the ongoing process of therapeutic development. In such an approach, the mind remains in a state of curiosity about process. Maintaining this open curiosity can be achieved only by reflectively using some of the interventions of a therapy on ourselves. Consequently, we gain an internal experience of therapeutic techniques, noting unexpected difficulties, fears, blocks, and resistances—and at times simply observing, "Oh, I didn't realize that." But equally important, with compassionate mind cultivation, we begin to observe the process of change, the strengthening and the development of the abilities to tolerate, to empathize, to feel grounded, to have a gentler orientation to the world, to deal with conflicts and setbacks in different ways, to tune into the fears behind self-criticism, and to replace them with a compassionate orientation to self and others. In addition, we develop a courageous dedication. Compassionate mind cultivation also enables us to feel more at peace and even joyful, living more mindfully, and appreciating and savoring the sensory complexity of the world around us.

This book is designed to help you learn compassionate mind training through genuine experience, which can create powerful shifts in how you approach life and work in the therapy room. In doing so, it invites you to think about a particular model of the human mind and a way of cultivating the mind so that you can approach life from a deeply compassionate orientation. It's a challenge. Compassion-focused therapy (CFT) is an integrative psychotherapy that utilizes many well-established therapeutic interventions—including thought and emotion monitoring, inference chaining, reappraisal, behavioral exposure, and rehearsal, to name just a few. You will meet these practices in the pages to come. When it comes to building, exploring, and cultivating a particular pattern we call the "compassionate self," you will engage in acting techniques that will prompt you to imagine what it would be like to be a deeply compassionate person, and how you would feel, think, and behave from this compassionate perspective. Compassionate mind training also shares many features found in Eastern contemplative traditions, such as mindfulness, groundedness, bodywork, and the cultivation of the compassionate self (in Buddhism, it's called *cultivating bodhicitta*). Personal practice with the determination to create a particular self-identity always walks hand in hand with the guidance of a guru or mentor. This book is designed to be a kind of self-explorative mentorship experience organized around processes of guided discovery, personal experimentation, practice, and reflection.

Building the compassionate self with the various practices you will encounter in this book is also intended to stimulate particular kinds of physiological patterns, such as those linked with the vagus nerve, the patterning of the autonomic nervous system, the frontal cortex, and oxytocin systems. This component is important because we use these physiological patterns to engage with things that are difficult or frightening. In CFT, we have a model that is designed to create the physiological pattern for compassion, which is an evolutionary-based regulator of threat processing. For example, children are biologically prepared to be soothed by the compassionate and kind signals they receive from the mother. So compassion itself offers a grounding experience such that if people do become overwhelmed or distressed, there is a safe and secure base to which to return. In addition, compassionate states have an impact on the frontal cortex, which allows individuals to have different insights that they wouldn't get necessarily through straight desensitization.

Compassion-Focused Therapy

The central focus of CFT is to address the essence of the human condition, which is the nature of suffering: how and why we suffer and what can we do about it (Gilbert, 2009, 2010, 2014). This was also the key pursuit of Siddhartha on his road to enlightenment and becoming a Buddha (which literally means *enlightened one*) over 2,500 years ago. Then, as now, the guidance was to look deeply into the nature of existence and its fluctuating and transient nature. In doing so, we become witness to the fact that we are all gene-directed biological short-lived beings who are born, grow, decay, and die. We are vulnerable to disease and injury in a world of high interdependence—for good and ill. In addition to these new and ancient insights into the nature of human existence, CFT rekindles some of the early psychodynamic questions—for instance, how does our understanding of ourselves as evolved biological beings impact the nature of our minds and our vulnerability to distress, and what do we do about the challenges this situation presents?

So this volume presents a quite personal, sometimes challenging entry into CFT. We need to spend time reflecting on our common humanity and what we are all caught up with, such as the fact that we have brains capable of fear, hate, yearning, love, and grief. We carry forward in time the history of mammalian life in our heads. From 2 million years ago, one of nature's primates began evolving a new range of competencies that gave us abilities for thinking, imagining, and a special kind of *knowing insight* and awareness that no other animal has. Nature gave birth to human minds. We are a consciousness that can become knowingly conscious of the contents of our own minds.

Whereas some therapies talk about how we fuse with our thoughts, CFT talks more about how we *con*fuse consciousness with content, and can even come to believe that we are defined by this content—this story of who we are—rather than understanding the self in terms of the awareness that can observe this story. Am I an angry person or am I a consciousness experiencing anger? Am I a traumatized person or am I consciousness experiencing the consequences of a brain responding to trauma?

The Buddhist scholar Matthieu Ricard has often said that a mind is like water; it can contain a poison or a medicine, but it *is* neither poison nor medicine, and it will become confused if it identifies with either. Mind is like a spotlight that can shine on many things, but is not defined by the things on which it shines. Taking an evolutionary approach helps people understand the nature of the contents of mind and helps them keep from overidentifying with any particular aspect of that content. Sometimes people can think of themselves as an "angry person" or a "traumatized person" or a "sad person . . . or a happy person . . . or a clever person . . . or a stupid person." However, these are all different labels for patterns of experience we may encounter or enact at different times but that ultimately do not define us. To paraphrase Daniel Siegel (2016), psychotherapy is a process of gradual differentiation as we begin to recognize these different processes within us without overidentification, allowing for integration that gives rise to transformation. In CFT, we see compassion as the main motivational process that allows this transformation to happen, because it facilitates turning toward and working with the difficulties of mind rather than overidentifying or fusing with them, avoiding them, or being overwhelmed by them. We begin to see mental states and mind states as patterns that lock us into states. This was very much a theme I tried to address in the book *Depression: From Psychology to Brain State* (Gilbert, 1984). So it's not just about changing behaviors, cognitions, beliefs, or emotions, although all of these can become a focus; CFT provides the context for radical change to arise by creating opportunities for the brain (especially now that we know about neuroplasticity and epigenetics) to organize itself into different patterns (Gilbert & Irons, 2005).

Understanding the Importance of Addressing the Dark Side

It is easy to get the impression that compassion is focused solely on being kind to ourselves and supportively and gently guiding ourselves through life. That's not a bad aim, and indeed cultivating friendliness, affiliation, and kind orientations toward ourselves and others can be extremely important. Such qualities build relationships, and the stimuli associated with kindness, such as vocal tone and facial expression, impact physiological structures such as the amygdala and the vagus nerve. Compassion, however, also requires that we build courage to address suffering. Indeed, we know that sometimes the most courageous people—for example, those who would rescue us from a burning house—may not be the kindest, and that the kindest people are not always the most courageous. For sure, compassion does not seek to act unkindly, but the emotions we experience depend upon the context. For example, entering the burning house to save a person or fighting against injustice wouldn't necessarily be regarded as kind but as compassionately courageous. Kindness, on the other hand, suggests the expression of a sentiment to others. It helps people experience us as safe, nonthreatening, and thoughtful, as caring about them in a particular way, suggesting that "we hold them in mind." Interestingly, if you ask people to show a compassionate facial expression, they will typically show a kind face with a gentle smile and smiling eyes (McEwan et al., 2014). However, facial expressions that involve smiling, however gentle, are not regarded as compassionate when one is in pain (Gerdes, Wieser, Alpers, Strack, & Pauli, 2012).

Compassion actually has a precise meaning: *sensitivity to suffering in self and others with a commitment to try to relieve and prevent it* (Gilbert, 2017a, 2017b). Like all motivations, we need to detect and respond to signals for that motive. So compassion competencies involve paying attention to and engaging with suffering rather than turning away or dissociating from it. Second, compassion involves making wise efforts to alleviate and prevent suffering rather than reacting impulsively or rashly to suffering. This book guides you in deepening your understanding of what compassion is and is not, and helps you develop the inner awareness and experiences that make compassion possible.

CFT recognizes the importance of also focusing on the dark side of mind: the aspects of mind that can drive despair into suicide, rage to murder, vengeance to torture, paranoia to hiding; a mind that can be in torment and can create torment for others. Compassion-focused therapists consider human minds in the context of evolution, as easily caught up and scripted by dramas driven by archetypal processes that helped our ancestors survive. Each of us is seeking to be loved, to belong, to be respected, to have satisfying sexual relationships, to have children who prosper, to live a long and healthy life—but equally to acquire the resources needed to overcome those who would threaten us. We want to relate to some people but not others, and we want to be related to by some people and not others. The mind comes ready-made with a whole set of needs, preferences and desires, wishes and wants that are choreographed by environments, for good and ill. This hardwiring of the human mind is why throughout history, humans have demonstrated capacities for wonderful achievements but also truly terrible, horrific actions. Compassion is one of our most courageous and dedicated motivations; it can help us do the difficult work of turning toward these darker aspects of our humanity and taking responsibility for working with them.

Nor is it easy for us to recognize that if we had been kidnapped as babies and raised in a violent drug gang, we would almost certainly now exist as very different versions of ourselves. Should this have happened to me, the current version of Paul Gilbert would not exist: My genetic expressions would be different, my brain architecture would be different, my values would be different, my preparedness to be violent would be different. So where is the *real* Paul Gilbert? This insight into our identities and the realization that there is no single "self" but only a varied set of biological patterns, greatly shaped by environmental contexts that texture our consciousness, is tricky for therapists. But it leads directly to the issue of why so much of what happens within us and between us is not our fault—*it's a setup*. This perspective also provides a very powerful orientation in therapy, because even if you're working with people who have done horrific things, it's important to remember that they are each a consciousness, textured by content around which they may have very little insight, and maybe even less control over. This point raises an interesting debate about free will, which space precludes us from pursuing here. But it also raises a very central element that is easily misunderstood: the greater the insight, the greater the responsibility. CFT is very much about building an ethical and moral orientation to the serious problems nature has given us in terms of the way our minds function. Indeed, as we begin to truly tune in to the reality of suffering and how endemic it is to human existence, we discover that compassion is the only response that makes any kind of sense. So compassion isn't just about addressing suffering in oneself and others, it's also about becoming increasingly motivated to *not* cause suffering intentionally, be it to yourself or others. So we shift from blaming and shaming to an enlightened ethic of taking responsibility, whenever we can, for our own behavior.

The compassion-focused therapist's road toward compassion involves developing the courage to engage with suffering and the causes of suffering, to genuinely stand up to say, "I will take responsibility for addressing suffering whenever I can." When we do this, we see that the causes of suffering arise because we are part of the flow of life, simply coming into existence, trying to survive, reproduce, and then going out of existence. Developing a deep inner connectedness to the flow of life profoundly affects how we work with ourselves and our clients, because we no longer see us or them as pathologically disturbed or simply bounced around by maladaptive schemas or attitudes (although we may be both). Rather, we see ourselves and others as struggling beings who didn't choose to be here, didn't choose this particular genetic architecture or its choreography in the dance of our personal lives, and didn't choose to suffer and struggle. When these pennies drop, people can begin to grow out of desires to be harmful to self through self-criticism or other ways. They can move from shame to a compassionate understanding that fuels the motivation to help.

Coming together in common humanity and recognizing that we are all part of the flow of life opens us to the reality that compassion is both an interpersonal and intrapersonal flow. There is the compassion we can cultivate *for* other people, but also our openness to receiving compassion *from* other people. Indeed, compassionate mind training is not just about self-compassion, but about cultivating these flows of compassion. There is research now showing that we can get into difficulties if we become overly self-reliant and either don't trust others or are fearful of allowing others to help us. Part of your journey isn't just developing compassion for yourself, but recognizing how the flow of compassion organizes your mind. When you are compassionate toward others, this compassion has an impact on your brain and how your mind is developing. When you are open, receptive, and responsive to the compassion of others, perhaps with a sense of gratitude, appreciation, or simply safeness because people around you were helpful, this open state will impact your brain and how your mind is developing. And, of course, when you are able to genuinely treat your own mind with empathic compassion, this will also have an impact on your brain and how your mind is developing. Following this path also means that you will need to address the many fears, blocks, and resistances that can impede these flows.

In a way, we can see compassion as a kind of field generator that is rippling through not just our minds but also the minds of others, creating patterns of consciousness through interconnectedness. Just as we can spread fear, prejudice, and hostility around us through how we act and the values we espouse, so we can create compassionate fields of consciousness. Our perspective can move beyond just what happens in our own heads as we begin to see ourselves as participants within an interpersonal field of mutually reciprocating influence (Siegel, 2016).

This Book

This book was inspired by the desire to help people interested in CFT use some of CFT's practices, insights, and philosophical orientations on themselves, and to see where it takes them. Rather than just reading about CFT with case examples and references, this book seeks to guide you into and through personal practice and reflections. This is no easy task, and these authors bring a wealth of experience to the journey. Russell Kolts, an author of several books on CFT and compassion, wanted to find ways of bringing the concepts of CFT to individuals in forensic settings and so developed the True Strength Program, applying CFT to the treatment of anger. He gained extraordinary insights into the ways in which individuals in prison, some of them for violent crimes, could develop a deep understanding of compassion and begin to walk that path of cultivating compassionate minds, once they overcame their resistances. This crucial shift began with their ability to understand compassion as a form of strength that gave them the courage to face the darkest parts of their lives and their minds.

Tobyn Bell, a very experienced clinician, supports training, runs CFT supervision groups, and is undertaking some fascinating PhD studies exploring the impact of some of the set practices, such as the multiple-selves exercises, on both clients and therapists. James Bennett-Levy has pioneered the use of self-practice and self-reflection in other therapies such as CBT and in some of the principles you will see here too. Chris Irons has many years of training in CFT, and we have copublished many articles and book chapters together. He is a very skilled clinician and runs therapy supervision groups in London and also self-practice compassionate mind training groups of personal development for the general public. All of the authors share this core desire to bring compassion to life through practice.

These very experienced CFT therapists will guide you through a number of the core concepts for developing insight into how our minds work and how we can begin to change patterns within them. You will learn ways to think about the evolutionary function of your motives and emotions in terms of their basic design and intent. This perspective will set you on the path to stand back from the contents of your mind, be they anger or anxiety, vengeance or self-criticism, and see these states as patterns of experience, separate from who you are. The question is whether you would like to continue or begin to change the pattern. If you wish to change the pattern, there are ways to do so. The four most important themes include developing specific capacities of mind, such as *mindfulness*—that is, becoming more attentive to what arises in you as it arises, but also learning to live more in the sensory world, appreciating the qualities of the senses. A second theme is *mind awareness*—beginning to understand why your mind does what it does, why it gets angry or anxious in the way that it does, or enjoys sexuality or a good bottle of wine! A third theme is *compassion*—learning about what compassion actually is (and is not) and the different competencies that support it, such as developing empathy, distress tolerance, different types of wisdom, and the practice of certain behaviors. You will also learn that CFT is not (just) about changing beliefs, but really focuses on creating a certain compassionate self-identity and practicing living from that identity. You can imagine that such an identity would organize your life very differently than would an identity constructed around the experience of anger. If every day you practiced cultivating your angry self to have more rage attacks in your life, and at every opportunity you practiced becoming irritated no matter how small the annoyance, then the result would be quite different. It would be a distinct contrast to the deliberate choice to live as your compassionate self, driven by qualities such as courage, wisdom, and the kind motivation to alleviate and prevent suffering and to address life's difficulties as best you could from that pattern of mind. A fourth theme is *intentionality*—how do we create compassionate intentions so that they are brought into action, moment by moment, into everyday life events and occurrences? How can we build our compassionate motivation and intention into the habits of daily living? There is increasing research that shows that if we build our intentions into habits, they stick. Indeed, we have data to show that when people start connecting with their compassionate selves in everyday life to work with particular difficulties, this can have a powerful effects, including upon heart rate variability (Matos et al., 2017). As you go through this book you will find many exercises, practice sheets, and opportunities for self-reflection on practices designed to help you build these compassion capacities into habits.

One of the core issues the authors discuss is preparing the body. We often use the motto *Respect the practice, prepare the body;* that is, use the body to support the mind. If your body is in a state of chaos, then it's difficult to hold your mind in a state of calm. Learning to ground your body with particular breathing techniques, postures, vocal tones, and facial expressions will help you in your orientation of compassion. This does not mean that compassion is always about grounding and soothing, because sometimes it involves acting out of fear, such as assertively addressing a problem or threat, or out of anger, as in fighting injustice. However, the practices offered here often involve grounding, and if you follow the ones outlined by these authors, you will begin to feel more grounded.

Finally, as these authors highlight, the journey into compassion is not necessarily one of wine and roses. It can be quite tough because you're going to be engaging with suffering. CFT makes a very clear distinction between safety and safeness. *Safety* is extremely important, but it's focused on the avoidance of potential harm. When you get into a car, you put on your safety belt; if you go mountain climbing, you ensure that your ropes are strong. If you go to the gym, staff will teach you how to use the equipment safely and not to start lifting weights that your muscles won't support. Safety is about harm prevention. Once harm has been minimized or prevented, we can focus on creating *safeness* in order to move forward to explore, develop, grow, and practice. It's exactly the same in therapy, or indeed in any kind of training. Before your journey, develop a clear intention in your mind to keep an eye on your pace and not engage in things that could be overwhelming to you until you're ready. Sometimes it's quite useful to do these practices with other people, so you might want to find some friends and go through the book together, sharing your experiences. But as the authors of this book make very clear, your journey with them is one of enlightenment, growth, and development, so try as best you can to keep that intention in mind, even if the road gets a little tricky at times. Ultimately, of course, for any personal practice, you'll need to take care of your own well-being.

All that remains for me now is to wish you well on your journey of exploration into the practices of compassion. Try to see this as the start of the journey. Imagine what your life would be like, and what you would be like as a therapist, if you deepened your ability to live from your inner, courageous, insightful, and compassionately wise self—or should I say *brain pattern*.

PAUL GILBERT, PhD, FBPsS, OBE

References

Ellenberger, H. F. (1970). *The discovery of the unconscious: The history and evolution of dynamic psychiatry.* New York: Basic Books.

Gerdes, A. B. M., Wieser, M. J., Alpers, G. W., Strack, F., & Pauli, P. (2012). Why do you smile at me while I'm in pain?: Pain selectively modulates voluntary facial muscle responses to happy faces. *International Journal of Psychophysiology, 85,* 161–167.

Gilbert, P. (1984). *Depression: From psychology to brain state.* Hove, UK: Erlbaum.

Gilbert, P. (2009). *The compassionate mind: A new approach to the challenge of life.* London: Constable & Robinson.

Gilbert, P. (2010). *Compassion focused therapy: Distinctive features.* London: Routledge.

Gilbert, P. (2014). The origins and nature of compassion focused therapy. *British Journal of Clinical Psychology, 53,* 6–41.

Gilbert, P. (2017a). Compassion: Definitions and controversies. In P. Gilbert (Ed.), *Compassion: Concepts, research and applications* (pp. 3–15). London: Routledge.

Gilbert, P. (2017b). Compassion as a social mentality: An evolutionary approach. In P.

Gilbert (Ed.), *Compassion: Concepts, research and applications* (pp. 31–68). London: Routledge.

Gilbert, P., & Irons, C. (2005). Focused therapies and compassionate mind training for shame and self-attacking. In P. Gilbert (Ed.), *Compassion: Conceptualisations, research and use in psychotherapy* (pp. 9–74). London: Routledge.

Matos, M., Duarte, C., Duarte, J., Pinto-Gouveia, J., Petrocchi, N., Basran, J., et al. (2017). Psychological and physiological effects of compassionate mind training: A pilot randomised controlled study. *Mindfulness, 8*(6), 1699–1712.

McEwan, K., Gilbert, P., Dandeneau, S., Lipka, S., Maratos, F., Paterson, K.B., et al. (2014). Facial expressions depicting compassionate and critical emotions: The development and validation of a new emotional face stimulus set. *PLoS ONE, 9*(2), e88783.

Siegel, D. J. (2016). *Mind: A journey to the heart of being human.* New York: Norton.

Contents

Purchasers of this book can download and print select forms at
www.guilford.com/kolts-forms (see copyright page for details).
The FOC scale can be found at
https://compassionatemind.co.uk/resources/scales.

Setting the Scene for CFT SP/SR

CHAPTER 1

Introducing *Experiencing Compassion-Focused Therapy from the Inside Out*

> If you want others to be happy, practice compassion.
> If you want to be happy, practice compassion.
> —His Holiness the 14th Dalai Lama

We (Russell, Tobyn, and Chris) were excited when James invited us to join him in creating a self-practice/self-reflection (SP/SR) book focused on compassion-focused therapy (CFT). A growing body of scientific research supports the value of compassion in working with mental health issues and in building happy lives, so naturally there is also a rapidly growing increase in clinicians who want to learn how to integrate compassion practices into their work with clients. Recent years have seen the development of resources to help therapists do just this. However, if you spend much time chatting with CFT therapists or others whose work focuses on compassion or mindfulness, you will hear them say time and time again, "If you're going to teach compassion or mindfulness, you need to practice it yourself." This statement conveys an increasing awareness—reflected in a growing body of scientific literature—that therapist SP/SR can deepen and enhance therapeutic work in a number of important ways across therapy models. The goal of this book is exactly that: to help you learn the fundamental experiences of CFT from the *inside out*, by cultivating, applying, and reflecting upon them in your own life.

A Brief Orientation to CFT

When you tell people that your area of therapist specialization is compassion-focused therapy, you're likely to get one of two reactions. The first (often spoken with raised eyebrows) is *"Compassion . . . that's nice. We all need more compassion, don't we?"* The second sort of response (often spoken in a really excited voice) sounds more like this: "Compassion-focused therapy! Me too! I've been doing that my *whole career*. Compassion is soooo important!" Both of these responses are based in the assumption that compassion-focused therapy, abbreviated *CFT,* simply involves doing therapy, well, *compassionately.*

Although embodying compassion in the therapy room certainly is a part of CFT (as we hope it would be in any therapy), it is much more than this. CFT was developed by Paul Gilbert in response to observations that many patients who struggled to benefit from traditional cognitive-behavioral therapy (CBT) approaches seemed to spend lots of time captured in patterns of shame and self-attacking. We can think of CFT as a "therapy model," but it's really more of an attempt to integrate what science tells us about what it means to be a human being, how and why we struggle, and how we can help people relate to their struggles in helpful, effective ways. In doing so, CFT draws heavily on multiple bodies of science as well as on wisdom traditions such as Buddhism. We draw from evolutionary psychology approaches in understanding the tricky ways that evolution has shaped our brains—ways that set us up for certain difficulties almost from the start. We draw from the evidence indicating that early attachment experiences can powerfully shape how we develop and how we learn to relate to ourselves and other people. We draw from affective neuroscience research that informs us about how our emotions and motives operate in our brains and minds, powerfully shaping our experience of life. We draw from behavioral and cognitive traditions that inform powerful technologies of change. And we also draw directly from traditions such as Buddhism, which have spent thousands of years exploring how practices of compassion and mindfulness can be cultivated in the service of building happy, healthy lives, communities, and civilizations (Gilbert, 2010).

Our Approach

A number of valuable books have been written on how these various influences are made manifest in CFT. The art of CFT involves bringing these influences alive in the form of basic human realizations and understandings, inspiring the courage our clients need to turn toward their struggles with kindness and commitment, and helping them cultivate a repertoire of compassionate strengths to draw upon in working with the inevitable challenges of having a human life. That's the focus of this book: not to tell you *about* CFT, but to bring CFT to life for you through your own experience of the therapy. You'll see all of these influences unfolding in the modules to come, in ways we hope will relate to both your personal and professional lives.

As we've already mentioned, the goal of this workbook is to give you an *experience* of practicing and reflecting upon the various ways that CFT seeks to help our clients develop compassion for themselves and others. As this process plays out, you'll be prompted to consider certain aspects of your experience and how your mind works. You'll also be asked to consider the ways in which you relate to yourself and to others, and how these strategies were shaped by your life experiences. You'll be exposed to a variety of compassion practices that you can try out in the context of your life. You'll then be given the opportunity to reflect upon these practices.

How This Book Is Organized

The next four chapters of *Experiencing Compassion-Focused Therapy from the Inside Out* prepare and orient you for the SP/SR modules in the rest of the book. Chapter 2 introduces some basic CFT concepts. It is not designed to be a comprehensive account—for that, you should read other books, such as those of Paul Gilbert (2009, 2010, 2014) and other CFT authors (e.g., Kolts, 2016; Welford, 2016; Irons & Beaumont, 2017). Rather, Chapter 2 provides a foretaste of some of the concepts introduced in the modules.

Chapter 3 provides the rationale and background for the SP/SR approach. It isn't necessary to read this chapter to use the book, but if you'd like to understand why we've chosen to design this book in a self-experiential way, you'll find the reasons here.

Chapter 4 is a long chapter, but an important one. We suggest that you read this chapter to get the most from the book. In the first half of the chapter, we discuss the pros and cons of the various contexts in which SP/SR can be undertaken—on your own, in a group, in "limited co-therapy pairs," in supervision, and in workshops. If you are doing SP/SR on your own, you can skip over the other contexts, but if you have the possibility to join with a colleague or group of colleagues to do SP/SR, the different ways that this can be done are worth considering. In the second half of Chapter 4, we suggest a variety of strategies, including creating a strong sense of safeness, to ensure you get the most benefit from SP/SR.

Chapter 5 is a brief chapter, but again an important one. It introduces you to your three "companion" therapists, whose self-practice exercises and self-reflections are peppered throughout the modules. All of these therapists struggle with issues we've adapted from our own experience as people and therapists, and those our colleagues have shared with us.

Following the opening five chapters are the SP/SR modules. These are purposely brief—designed to take you about 30–45 minutes apiece—in which you'll have the opportunity to work from the inside out, seeing how various CFT practices are applied by your companion therapists, and then trying them out yourself. You may find that you don't have time to do all the modules. Chapter 4 provides some suggestions for selecting modules if you only have limited time.

In preparing for SP/SR, you might consider issues in your professional or personal life to which bringing compassion might be of value: For instance, there may be contexts in which you tend to experience shame, criticize yourself, experience threatening emotions, or perhaps just have a lack of confidence. The point is to highlight an area of struggle or difficulty in your life that you can turn toward with courage, kindness, and a compassionate commitment to help.

It's also important to keep in mind that with SP/SR, the purpose is to use the approach with ourselves as a vehicle for learning the therapy, so that we can better serve our clients. In this way, it might be useful for you to choose an issue that relates to your work with clients. This also means that whereas you want to choose an issue that is substantive enough for you to "get" the processes involved, you don't want to choose a severe problem that can activate intense levels of distress in you, such as very recent and intense grief experiences. Chapter 4 will help you to select an issue which will work best in the context of this SP/SR workbook.

CHAPTER 2

A Brief Roadmap to CFT

Defining Compassion

Just as there is sometimes confusion about what CFT is, there can also be a lack of clarity about what is meant by the word *compassion.* In this book, we work from the standard definition used in CFT: sensitivity to suffering in self and others combined with the commitment to try to alleviate and prevent it (Gilbert & Choden, 2013). This definition contains two fundamental components, or as Paul Gilbert says, two "psychologies of compassion." The first is *sensitivity and engagement:* that is, the ability to notice, attend to, and be moved by suffering, as well as the willingness to *turn toward the suffering,* tolerate the distress associated with doing so, and look deeply into the causes and conditions that maintain it. Once we are aware of this suffering and experience a sympathetic response to the person who is suffering, this sensitivity can give rise to the *motivation and commitment* to act to alleviate current suffering in the self and others, and to prevent it in the future. This motivation and commitment contains both a felt desire to work to address the suffering, as well as the conscious decision and the skills required to do so.

In considering this definition of compassion, it's important to note that it contains both kindness and courage; at its heart, compassion is defined by the courageous willingness to *approach* the things that scare us and make us uncomfortable—about the world, and about ourselves (Gilbert, 2015). This compassionate approach is defined by the motive to help and characterized by caring, warmth, and commitment rather than judgment and condemnation. For many of our clients (and ourselves) this simple definition represents a very different way of relating to our ourselves and to suffering, particularly if we've learned to criticize ourselves when we see ourselves struggling, or to manage difficult emotions by avoiding them or distracting ourselves from pain or discomfort when we become aware of it.

CFT practitioners also commonly talk about three *flows* of compassion: the compassion we direct from ourselves to others, the compassion we receive from other people, and the compassion we direct toward ourselves. Recent research has shown that these different flows seem to work in somewhat different ways (Gilbert et al., 2017), which raises the likelihood that one may be very high in one form of compassion, but struggle greatly with another form. For example, most therapists have great compassion for their clients, but some may be virtually unable to allow themselves to feel vulnerable in receiving it from others, or to relate compassionately to themselves when they need it.

Cultivating Compassion: The CFT Perspective

In CFT, compassion is seen as being rooted in *motivation*—the motivation to alleviate and prevent suffering (Gilbert, 2015). This experience begins with an awareness of what it means to have a human life in this day and age. The idea is that once we take a deep look at the reality of what it means to have a human life—the amount of struggle and difficulty we all face eventually as a result of simply being born human—*compassion is the only response that makes sense* (Gilbert, 2009). If we look at the life of even a relatively privileged human being—someone who has regular access to food, shelter, health care, education, and caring relatives and friends—we can see almost countless sources of pain and potential suffering. We will all get sick. We will all eventually die. Along the way, we will lose people we love, will try our best and fail, and will face disappointment, tragedy, and struggle time and time again. And depending on the conditions of our birth—whether we were born with a hearty or vulnerable body, and whether we were born to people who were (or were not) capable of caring for us in ways that helped us grow up happy and healthy—some of us will face considerably more pain and struggle.

Some readers may be surprised to learn that in CFT, we don't immediately start out with the compassion meditations. We've found that for individuals with deeply entrenched habits of shame and self-criticism, promoting compassion (and self-compassion, in particular) can be very tricky, sometimes even stimulating feelings of threat. For some of us, even thinking about treating ourselves with compassion and kindness (or being treated this way by others) can be very scary and contrary to how we've learned to exist in the world. In CFT, efforts have been made to assess and explore these "fears of compassion" (Gilbert, McEwan, Matos, & Rivis, 2011), which have been linked with depression, anxiety, alexithymia, and insecure attachment styles (Gilbert, McEwan, Catarino, Baião, & Palmeira, 2014).

For this reason, CFT involves "preparing the ground" by helping ourselves and our clients gain certain realizations about what it means to have a human life—realizations that can soften the coarse ground of shame and self-criticism so that the seeds of self-compassion can take root and grow. Many of these realizations have to do with the challenges presented by our evolved brain systems and the social shaping we've received, particularly in our earliest environments. With such reflection, we can begin to become aware that many of our struggles are rooted in factors that we didn't get to choose or design, and it can be liberating to realize that *they are not our fault*. In CFT, we emphasize recognizing the unchosen factors that have shaped us in ways we wouldn't have chosen, so we can stop beating ourselves up for things that aren't our fault and take responsibility for working actively and effectively to improve our lives in the present and in the future.

In this perspective, CFT emphasizes the cultivation of mindful, accepting awareness, so we can learn to observe the thoughts, emotions, and experiences that define our struggles without judgment. This awareness then leads to another core component of CFT: learning to directly cultivate compassion in order to alleviate and prevent suffering in ourselves and others. In this book, you'll gain experience with a number of compassion practices—some shared with other approaches and some unique to CFT—that will help you do just that.

In summary, we can consider the process of CFT as one in which we work to develop a number of compassionate capacities. We want to build the caring *motivation* and *courage* to work directly with the sources of suffering in our lives. We want to develop the *wisdom* to understand the sources of this suffering, rooted in the intersection between our biological inheritance and our life experiences. We want to cultivate a discerning *awareness* of how this suffering plays out in our lives and in our mental experiences. And finally, we want to engage in committed *compassionate action* to work with this suffering and its causes.

Preparing the Ground for Compassion

Although there are a number of programs aimed at helping people to cultivate compassion in their lives—most notably Neff and Germer's mindful self-compassion program (Germer & Neff, 2017) and Stanford's compassion cultivation training (Jazaieri et al., 2013)—CFT is the only *model of psychotherapy* with an explicit focus on compassion. Whereas these other models focus primarily on compassion cultivation practices adapted from Buddhist compassion meditations (which CFT utilizes as well), as mentioned above, CFT also includes an explicit focus on helping clients develop an inherently de-shaming way of understanding the human experience. One way of doing this is by helping clients understand their experience in the context of how evolution has shaped human brains, and through this, shaped our basic motives and emotional functioning in ways that can sometimes be tricky to manage. A core realization in CFT is that our emotions and motivations aren't something that are wrong with us, but are products of brains that evolved to help our ancestors survive in a world that was very different from the one we currently face. In our ancestors' world in which most threats were physical in nature, the felt urgency and pure focus of threat-related emotions such as fear, anxiety, and anger made a lot of sense—even as they're a poor fit with most of the difficult situations we face in modern life.

In going through the experiential modules in this book, you'll become familiar with a number of these concepts, including the tricky interactions between our "old brains," which are guided by basic motives and produce powerful emotions, and our "new brains," which are very sophisticated in their ability to assign meaning and create nuanced thinking and imagery, but which can be harnessed by our emotions in ways that can create problems for us (e.g., through generating the sorts of ruminative thinking that can fuel ongoing anxiety). You'll also explore the "three circles" model of motivation and emotion, in which clients learn to understand their emotions and basic motives—many of which they may struggle with or criticize themselves for having—through the lens of evolutionary function. In this model, emotions are organized into three systems. The first is the threat and self-protection system ("threat system" for short), which produces emotions (e.g., anger, fear) and motives organized around detecting and responding to perceived threats, and has a narrowing effect upon our attention, thinking, and motivational processes. The second system is the drive and resource acquisition system ("drive system"), responsible for motivating us to focus on and pursue goals, and rewarding us for attaining them. Finally, there is the safeness and soothing system ("safeness system"), which is linked with experiences of feeling safe, content, calm, and peaceful, and in humans tends to be linked with nurturing and affiliative experiences. This system is underpinned by the parasympathetic nervous system and is focused upon in CFT as a way to balance out experiences of threat and pave the way for compassion, as it is associated with attentional flexibility, reflective thinking, and prosocial tendencies (Gilbert, 2009, 2010).

When clients can understand the emotions they struggle with as their evolved brain's attempts to protect them, their shame can soften. As you'll learn, CFT also helps clients explore how their current lives are related to various socially shaping experiences they've had, as a way to better understand how their struggles make perfect sense when considered within the developmental context of their lives. Although the rest of this book is focused on an experiential exploration of these and other concepts, there are a number of resources available for readers who would like to spend more time exploring the theoretical foundations of CFT (e.g., Gilbert, 2009, 2010; Kolts, 2016; Welford, 2016; Irons & Beaumont, 2017).

CHAPTER 3

Why Do SP/SR?

⁂

There are many competing demands on busy therapists' time. As a prospective SP/SR participant, you may be wondering if it's worth the investment of precious personal time and resources to do a CFT SP/SR program. What can SP/SR do that can't be done through other means of learning—reading a CFT textbook, going to a workshop, or seeking supervision? What are the benefits of SP/SR, and what are the costs?

These questions are the focus of the next two chapters. In this chapter, we begin by examining the qualities we seek to develop as CFT therapists. We then consider the value of personal practice for CFT therapists and spend a bit of time reviewing the evidence for SP/SR. We'll also address the question of how SP/SR can contribute to the development of CFT therapist qualities and skills. Considering the evidence in support of SP/SR, we suggest that CFT SP/SR may play an important and perhaps unique role in the CFT therapist's personal and professional development. And then in Chapter 4, "Getting the Most from SP/SR," we provide concrete recommendations designed to help you get the most from the program.

Qualities of the CFT Therapist

In common with other therapies, CFT therapists need a good understanding of their particular model—an understanding of both the conceptual aspects (e.g., the evolutionary model, three circles) and the technical aspects (e.g., CFT imagery practices, compassionate letter writing). CFT therapists also require the ability to translate this understanding into procedural skills-in-action for use with clients, combining them effectively with interpersonal skills such as empathy, compassion, and therapeutic presence.

As with other therapies, CFT also recognizes the central importance of a therapeutic relationship characterized by the Rogerian attributes of empathy, warmth, and genuineness (Rogers, 1951). However, CFT also emphasizes two other therapist attributes that are central to the particular way we work (Kolts, 2016):

1. CFT therapists aim to create the conditions that will facilitate a *secure attachment relationship* with their clients.
2. CFT therapists should *model the flow of compassion*—compassion for other, capacity to receive compassion, and self-compassion.

Secure Attachment Relationships

All therapies are relational by their very nature. However, the focus and type of therapeutic relationship differ to some extent across different therapies (e.g., psychoanalysis, CBT, schema therapy, CFT). In the case of CFT, the creation of a sense of safeness in the therapeutic relationship is considered to be of prime importance (Gilbert, 2014). Fostering this sense of safeness can be tricky, because many clients may have very rarely experienced feelings of safeness in their relationships. Creating that sense of safeness and asking clients to reflect on how they experience it can set the stage for compassion by helping them learn to regulate experiences of threat, balance their emotions, and connect with their compassionate intention to engage with suffering rather than avoid it.

Attachment theory provides a theoretical framework to help CFT therapists understand their role in creating a sense of safeness (Bowlby, 1988). A number of studies now suggest that the attachment style of the therapist has a direct impact on therapeutic outcome (Berry & Danquah, 2016; Black, Hardy, Turpin, & Parry, 2005; Mikulincer, Shaver, & Berant, 2013). Therapists who are anxiously attached or avoidant have poorer client outcomes than therapists who are securely attached. Therefore, it behooves CFT therapists to reflect upon their own attachment style, and if needed, work toward developing their therapeutic presence in order to provide a secure base for their clients. Modules 10 and 31 have been included to enable participants to consider their attachment style and how this style may affect their relationships with clients.

Modeling the Flow of Compassion

Since therapists' sensitivity to suffering, compassionate motivation, and compassionate action are core to the development of compassion skills in clients, it is also important for CFT therapists to model a compassionate presence for clients. We suspect that most therapists already have a strong compassion-for-other motivation, which likely has a lot to do with why they chose to become therapists. However, recent research indicates that many therapists have relatively poor self-compassion skills (Finlay-Jones, Rees, & Kane, 2015; Raab, 2014). For instance, on the Young Schema Scale, unrelenting standards and self-sacrifice are the two most frequently endorsed schemas (Haarhoff, 2006; Kaeding et al., 2017). Therapists who implicitly or explicitly model self-criticism, self-sacrifice, and perfectionistic habits may be less than optimal models for highly self-critical clients.

Furthermore, these attributes may contribute significantly to stress and burnout, with considerable personal cost and reduction in therapeutic effectiveness (Patsiopoulos & Buchanan, 2011; Raab, 2014; Kaeding et al., 2017). In contrast, treating ourselves *and* our clients with compassion can create a powerful model of self-care for clients and enable us to function more effectively as people and therapists.

For all the above reasons, being attuned to the client's fluctuations on a moment-by-moment basis during sessions is particularly important for the CFT therapist. This attunement requires therapists to attend and respond mindfully to clients in the moment—what Schön (1983) termed "reflection-in-action." In remaining mindful, therapists need to maintain awareness of both their "personal self" (e.g., "What emotions am I experiencing right now?"; "Is my threat system being activated?") and their "therapist self" (e.g., "How can I best conceptualize my client's difficulties?"; "Can I use my threat reactions to understand what is going on in the relationship?") (Bennett-Levy & Haarhoff, in press). And like other therapists, CFT therapists will benefit from developing their capacity to use self-reflection between sessions—"reflection-on-action" (Schön, 1983)—to be maximally effective (Bennett-Levy, 2006; Rønnestad & Skovholt, 2003).

What Do CFT Therapists Say about Personal Practice?

To date, there has been just one study that has reported the impact of personal practice for CFT therapists (Gale, Schröder, & Gilbert, 2017). Gale et al. interviewed 10 CFT therapists about their experiences of personal practice during and after training. The study does not report how much personal practice the participants engaged in, or of what kind, except that two had attended a CFT personal practice workshop, and that most were actively receiving CFT supervision. Although presumably none of the participants were engaged in a formal SP/SR process—there were no SP/SR workbooks or SP/SR groups at that stage—the reported outcomes bear striking similarities to previous SP/SR research discussed in the next section. Gale et al. (2017) concluded:

> Personal practice of CFT can increase understanding of the approach, and confidence in using the approach. It can help therapists to anticipate difficulties clients may encounter and identify ways of overcoming these. It can also help to increase compassion for the self and for others, and impact on the therapeutic stance. Thus, personal practice of CFT can help to develop and refine therapeutic skills, but it could also be helpful as a self-care strategy for therapists. (p. 184)

With regard to the desirable qualities of CFT therapists outlined in the previous section, it is of particular interest that participants reported that personal practice of CFT increased their compassion for both self and others. Other data in the Gale et al. study indicated that personal practice increased self-awareness, suggesting the value of therapists using SP/SR to examine their attachment styles. For instance, one participant reported:

"I think CFT has definitely made me think more about what I bring as a therapist, really, to therapy and to the people I am working with. . . . Developing and doing self-practice is about going into those parts of yourself as well, which can be difficult and painful."

In common with other SP/SR studies, Gale et al. (2017) reported that personal practice of CFT enhanced both declarative understandings of the model and procedural skills-in-action. For instance, one participant said, "I think it really helped me get to grips with the model and also how you'd use the model with people" (p. 181). The participant also noted the importance of reflection, combined with personal practice.

A particularly interesting feature of Gale et al.'s (2017) findings was the observation that personal practice of CFT was not just a way to embed therapist skills or work on some personal issue. Personal practice of CFT impacted participants at a core level; compassion had become "a way of life" in therapists' personal and professional lives. As one participant remarked, "It feels very different to other therapies in that it is not just something that you use at work but almost like a philosophy that you hold about life generally" (p. 181).

SP/SR Research

SP/SR was initially developed as a training strategy to enhance the development of therapists' skills through practicing therapy strategies on themselves and reflecting on the experience, first from a personal perspective and then from a professional perspective (Bennett-Levy et al., 2001). Although the primary focus of SP/SR was initially on developing and refining CBT skills, the SP/SR protocol can easily be applied to any therapy that is amenable to self-practice. As noted in the preceding section, it has also become increasingly clear that SP/SR participants often experience personal as well as professional benefits (Bennett-Levy & Haarhoff, in press; Bennett-Levy, Thwaites, Haarhoff, & Perry, 2015; Pakenham, 2015). For instance, SP/SR can be used to address personal or professional issues or enhance therapist self-care.

SP/SR has been offered in two forms: as a workbook to be undertaken individually (Bennett-Levy et al., 2001; Davis, Thwaites, Freeston, & Bennett-Levy, 2015; Haarhoff, Gibson, & Flett, 2011), and in "limited co-therapy pairs" (Bennett-Levy, Lee, Travers, Pohlman, & Hamernik, 2003; Sanders & Bennett-Levy, 2010), in which each partner has the opportunity to be "therapist" and "client" (see Chapter 4 for further details). There is value in each of these forms (Thwaites, Bennett-Levy, Davis, & Chaddock, 2014). However, as we suggest in Chapter 4, there may be some advantages in the limited co-therapy form for CFT therapists, since this allows participants to experience the impact of compassion from another firsthand.

Figure 3.1, based on a model of SP/SR in Bennett-Levy and Finlay-Jones (in press), illustrates how we anticipate CFT SP/SR practice is likely to impact participants.

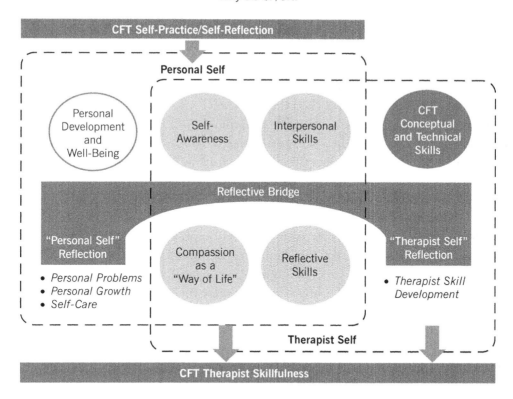

FIGURE 3.1. Model of the impact of SP/SR on CFT skills.

Research suggests that a primary impact of SP/SR is on therapists' self-awareness and interpersonal skills (Bennett-Levy & Finlay-Jones, in press; Thwaites et al., 2014; Thwaites et al., 2017). Typically, therapists engaging in SP/SR report enhanced mindful awareness of their internal processes (physical feelings, emotions, thoughts), and sometimes significant insights about underlying processes (e.g., their fears or reluctance to engage in a practice of compassion).

SP/SR participants also consistently report a primary impact on interpersonal skills such as empathic understanding and attunement, therapeutic presence, and compassion (Gale & Schröder, 2014; Spendelow & Butler, 2016; Thwaites et al., 2014). Typically, they make the link between their own experience of struggling with emotions or difficulty making changes with how it must be for the client:

> "It [SP/SR] was extremely valuable, both personally and professionally. I don't know . . . how you can have any understanding or be able to anticipate what people are going to go through or what their own resistances and dilemmas might be if you're not prepared to do that yourself."

Research also indicates that SP/SR enhances therapists' conceptual and technical skills (Gale & Schröder, 2014; Thwaites et al., 2014). A difference between SP/SR and personal therapy is that the learning from personal therapy is usually focused largely or completely on the personal self (e.g., addressing personal problems or personal growth). In contrast, although the self-experiential nature of SP/SR means that it begins with reflection on the personal self, SP/SR seeks to build an explicit "reflective bridge" between the "personal self" and the "therapist self" via reflective questions (Bennett-Levy & Haarhoff, in press; Bennett-Levy & Finlay-Jones, in press). It is by making this bridge and by experiencing the conceptual and technical aspects of CFT for yourself that SP/SR can enhance your conceptual and technical CFT skills.

To create a reflective bridge, SP/SR reflective questions usually follow a structured sequence; they focus first on the personal self ("What was your experience of self-practice?"; "How do you understand that experience?") and then bridge to the therapist self ("What are the implications for your therapeutic practice?"; "What are the implications for your understanding of CFT theory?") (Bennett-Levy et al., 2015; Thwaites et al., 2014). For instance, if we practice compassionate-self imagery, we not only start to develop the compassionate self, but we also consider the implications of our experience for how we introduce compassionate-self imagery to our clients.

In summary, there is now a body of SP/SR research that supports SP/SR as an effective training strategy that integrates the declarative with the procedural, the interpersonal with the technical and conceptual, and the personal self with the therapist self. Self-awareness and self-reflection provide the glue that enables the personal self to inform and influence the therapist self and to facilitate the effective blending of different therapy skills with one another. SP/SR participants tend to report major shifts in their appreciation of the therapeutic process, and in the ways that they engage with clients. In particular, through their own experience, participants report becoming much more aware of potential blocks to therapeutic progress, and consequently they become more effective at anticipating, noticing, and addressing those blocks.

The Value of SP/SR for CFT Therapists

To return to where we started, creating safeness in the therapeutic relationship and modeling compassionate ways of relating toward both self and others are central elements in CFT. Self-awareness and sophisticated interpersonal skills are key elements in embodying compassion and creating safeness—and each is enhanced by personal practice. In turn, self-awareness and interpersonal skills need to be well integrated with CFT conceptual and technical skills to facilitate the provision of effective CFT therapy. SP/SR assists this integration through the creation of a reflective bridge between the personal self and the therapist self.

We'd like to suggest that personal practice in the form of SP/SR makes an important—and perhaps unique—contribution to CFT therapist development. It is worth stopping to ask, "What other training or professional development strategies enhance self-awareness and interpersonal skills and provide a bridge between the personal and the professional domains?" Reading? Lectures or discussion? Modeling? Role play? A 2009 study reported that self-experiential learning and reflective practice were rated as more useful strategies for the development of interpersonal and reflective skills than were didactic learning, modeling, or role play (Bennett-Levy, McManus, et al., 2009). When experiential learning and reflective practice are provided in the form of SP/SR, the process enables participants to integrate these skills with conceptual and technical skills.

For therapists, time is a precious resource; professional development decisions should be made wisely. SP/SR is different from typical training strategies in that it makes significant emotional as well as intellectual demands on participants. SP/SR demands commitment, time, and energy. The benefit for SP/SR participants is that the emotional demands may lead to enhanced self-care and personal development as well as to the enhancement of therapist skills. For CFT therapists who are ready to take this step, SP/SR may provide unique insights, skills, and rich rewards for both professional and personal development. As we emphasize in Chapter 4, prospective SP/SR participants should consider the best time for them to take part in an SP/SR program, with whom, and under what conditions. Chapter 4 provides guidance in making these choices to maximize the benefits of SP/SR.

CHAPTER 4

Getting the Most from SP/SR

The purpose of this chapter is to help create an enriching experience of CFT SP/SR so that you gain the maximum benefit, both professionally and personally. The chapter is divided into two sections. In the first section, we look at some of the different contexts in which *Experiencing Compassion-Focused Therapy from the Inside Out* can be used—individually, in pairs, in groups, in supervision, and in workshops—and how to use these contexts to best effect. In the second section, we discuss important elements to consider for your SP/SR program so that it works as well for you as possible (e.g., creating a sense of safeness, time management, written reflections, choice of modules).

Different Contexts for SP/SR

Because the number of university-accredited CFT programs is currently very limited, we imagine that most readers will be creating their own contexts for doing CFT SP/SR. Deciding which context might work best for you and creating a helpful structure around it are two of the keys to a successful program. Here we consider how best to establish a flourishing SP/SR program in different contexts.

Doing SP/SR Individually

We anticipate that the majority of therapists using this book will choose to do the program individually. In many ways, this is the simplest option, and there are a number of advantages. You can start when you want, take as long as you want, personalize your program, and choose the modules that most appeal to you. You can build your personal and professional skills over time. Furthermore, without the constraint of anyone else being involved, some people feel freer to go deeper in their self-exploration. You don't have to worry about feeling exposed or embarrassed, and you don't need to negotiate confidentiality agreements with other people. However, if you decide to do the program on your own, you'll need to maintain a fairly high level of organization and self-discipline, as it's easy to put the workbook down for a couple of weeks and then fail to pick it up again. See the section on time management later in this chapter for some tips on working with these tendencies.

There are two disadvantages to doing SP/SR on your own; if you are aware of them, you can compensate for them to some extent. The first is that you don't get to experience two of the three flows of compassion directly within the SP/SR program; that is, you'll focus a great deal on self-compassion, but you'll miss out on giving compassion to others and receiving compassion from others. Therefore, we suggest that you may compensate for these missing components by focusing explicitly on giving and receiving compassion in between SP/SR sessions. The second disadvantage is that you don't get to experience the reflections of others. Different people experience therapeutic processes in different ways, and sometimes practices that don't work well for you may be quite powerful for others, and vice versa. Hearing or reading the reflections of others makes this very clear. Therefore we suggest that it is worth considering teaming up with a colleague in a limited co-therapy pair or forming an SP/SR group (see the next sections). However, neither option may be possible, and the great benefit of doing SP/SR on your own is that you have full control of your timetable, choice of modules, and the pace of your program.

SP/SR Groups

We explore various aspects of SP/SR groups in specific sections later in the chapter. Here we begin by highlighting some key elements of group approaches to SP/SR:

- Online or face-to-face SP/SR groups are often combined with individual "practice" or "practice occurring within" co-therapy pairs.
- SP/SR participants report groups to be one of most valuable aspects of SP/SR programs.
- A particular benefit of groups is that they enable participants to compare and contrast their experience of CFT practices with others, and to see that "one size does not fit all"—that people have a variety of reactions.
- Group participants may learn better reflective skills through experiencing the reflective writings and verbal reflections of others.
- Groups can function as supportive "learning communities" or "communities of practice"; at best, learning within groups can provide a far richer experience than individual learning.

There are various kinds of groups: groups within accredited CFT training programs, supervision groups, peer groups, groups of work colleagues, and facilitated online groups, to name but a few. Ground rules will vary depending on the type of relationships within these groups; for instance, some groups may meet face-to-face regularly; others may meet online; and others may never meet, except through their written reflections. With all groups, it's important to hold one or two preprogram meetings to clarify the process, address all participants' concerns around safeness and process, and reach clear agreements that are then written up and circulated to everyone.

Limited Co-Therapy Pairs

A less commonly reported form of SP/SR involves the formation of limited co-therapy pairs (Bennett-Levy et al., 2003; Sanders & Bennett-Levy, 2010). In this form of SP/SR, pairs of therapists essentially swap therapy sessions, with one member functioning as the therapist and the other as the client. In this context, the "client" works on a particular issue and the therapist works to facilitate the client's process, drawing upon the therapy techniques and strategies presented in the book. Then the two verbally reflect on their experiences as therapist and client. After a break, perhaps for a cup of tea or coffee, the pair swaps roles and repeats the process. Following their session, each writes up and shares his or her written reflections, which are discussed either online or perhaps at the start of the following session.

Limited co-therapy pairs involve personal sharing and therefore require a trusting relationship. This form of SP/SR is the closest approximation to the therapy context, and as such, involves greater levels of vulnerability for the participants. The payoff is that for some people, having a "limited co-therapist" may lead to some surprising insights and deeper exploration than could be achieved by working individually.

Arguably the co-therapy format is more personally challenging—but perhaps particularly well suited to CFT SP/SR. As we mentioned above, the co-therapy format enables people to experience and reflect upon each of the three flows of compassion (giving, receiving, and self-compassion), whereas the individual SP/SR format allows only a direct experience of self-compassion.

Because of the potential benefits of limited co-therapy, and because this interpersonal form of SP/SR may be particularly valuable for CFT, we suggest that, where possible, CFT therapists should be courageous! Take the risk and consider teaming up with another therapist, or group of therapists, to create a co-therapy pair or group of pairs, as in the Bennett-Levy et al. (2003) study. However, a brief word of caution: Pair up with a therapist in whose skills you have some confidence. As you'll see later in this chapter, it's helpful to be aware that good Socratic questions from your "therapist" can sometimes lead you to unexpectedly challenging places.

Limited co-therapy also involves considering some pragmatic concerns, such as allowing for enough time. Typically, you might allow 45 minutes for a session, then reflect for 10 minutes, then take a break before the changeover, then repeat the process.

With written reflections between sessions, and reflection on these written reflections, the process can be time-consuming—but very valuable.

An alternative to limited co-therapy may be to team up with someone else for specific exercises. This could be an interesting alternative to individual SP/SR for groups that meet face-to-face. As you go through the book, you'll see some modules that feature examples of therapists working together dyadically. Some CFT strategies are also particularly amenable to dyadic work (e.g., multiple selves). When you do have an opportunity to participate in limited co-therapy or dyadic exercises together, we would encourage you to do so.

SP/SR in Supervision

SP/SR can be a very useful adjunct to supervision. Some supervisees value the opportunity to work through experiential exercises, such as those in this workbook, between sessions and reflect on their experience with their supervisor. Alternatively, they may decide that a good way to embed their CFT skills is to try out specific strategies with their supervisor in a limited co-therapy role during sessions. In either case, it is important that the supervisor has had training in CFT as well as supervision in his or her own practice of CFT. There should also be a clear agreement for personal experiential work to be an explicit part of the supervision contract.

Supervision is a wonderful opportunity for supervisees not only to learn CFT skills, but also to experience the flow of compassion by receiving it from the supervisor. One of the later modules in this workbook (Module 32) focuses on the development of the "internal compassionate supervisor." For supervisors and supervisees alike, this is a valuable module, in which you consider and engage with the qualities of your ideal compassionate supervisor, which may then be used to work with difficult experiences in therapy.

As with other forms of SP/SR, we suggest that written reflections should play a role in the supervisory process. Supervisors might consider whether these reflections should be two-way, including not only reflections of the supervisee, but also those of the supervisor.

SP/SR in Workshops

Self-experiential exercises are sometimes part of training workshops. These may be one-off exercises or a series of connected exercises (Haarhoff & Thwaites, 2016). Our experience is that usually such exercises are debriefed verbally in pair or group format. However, we have also experimented with using written reflections in workshops for 3–5 minutes prior to the verbal debrief. When we have done so, the benefits seem rich, deepening the experience of the participants and creating a different atmosphere and pace to the workshop—a pace in which reflection can flourish.

Essential Elements in SP/SR Programs

Creating a Sense of Safeness

As we have seen, creating a sense of safeness is a fundamental element of CFT. Research shows that the experience of safeness is a key requirement for an SP/SR program as well (Bennett-Levy & Lee, 2014; Spafford & Haarhoff, 2015). Whether you are doing SP/SR individually or in a group, safeness matters.

Research on SP/SR programs indicates that there are two fears related to safeness that need to be addressed for SP/SR participants to engage fully: fear that SP/SR may lead to loss of control or personal distress, and fear of exposure to other participants in group situations (Bennett-Levy & Lee, 2014). Both fears should be addressed before starting an SP/SR program. As we illustrate in the following sections, there are numerous strategies that have been developed with precisely this purpose in mind.

Creating Safeness and a Sense of Control within the SP/SR Process

Fear that SP/SR may lead to loss of control or personal distress can be addressed in several ways. Firstly, as an SP/SR participant, you have control over the issue(s) that you choose to focus on and the depth at which you do any particular exercise. It is recommended that the issue you select should be at an emotional intensity range of not less than 40% on a scale where 100% equals maximum distress (otherwise it is unlikely to sustain you over the program), and ideally 50–75%—definitely no more than 80%. A degree of discomfort is expected from SP/SR, which in itself provides an opportunity for self-compassion (Gilbert & Irons, 2005; Germer & Neff, 2013). However, if you find an exercise to be overactivating, use it as an opportunity to bring compassion to yourself by touching on it only lightly—or maybe not at all.

Secondly, there are some issues which should be avoided in SP/SR programs—in particular, issues linked to trauma or abuse, high levels of grief, very distressing memories, or a current major life issue (e.g., a relationship breakup). Additionally, if you are currently experiencing high levels of stress at work or home, this might not be the best time to undertake an SP/SR program (Bennett-Levy et al., 2001).

Thirdly, occasionally one thing leads to another, and participants can be taken by surprise by the intensity of feelings and memories aroused by a particular exercise. Just as we might suggest that our clients use various compassionate mind training strategies (e.g., soothing rhythm breathing, safe place imagery) to help regulate their threat system reactions, under these circumstances, we should do similarly. Even then, there are times when troubling memories may persist. When this happens, it may be wise to seek external support. For this reason, we suggest that everyone creates for him- or herself a Personal Safeguard Strategy. Typically, a Personal Safeguard Strategy has at least three levels, including identifying a potential therapist before an SP/SR program actually starts. For instance:

- Level 1: Talk with your partner, good friend, or a trusted colleague.
- Level 2: Discuss the issue with your supervisor; create a plan.
- Level 3: Make appointment with a trusted therapist.

Creating Safeness in SP/SR Groups

We're anticipating that some participants may choose to do the SP/SR program in a group setting. For these individuals, addressing participants' fears of exposure to others will be key to creating safeness. When participants first consider doing SP/SR in a group format, it is natural that a primary concern is confidentiality. This and other concerns around safeness need to be addressed before the program starts. For this reason, the SP/SR protocol is that any potential SP/SR group should have the opportunity to meet on one or two occasions before beginning the program. All issues and concerns should be aired (e.g., confidentiality, program timelines, expectations, requirements), and strategies developed to address these (Bennett-Levy et al., 2015). Once developed, agreements should be written down and circulated. For further ideas about preprogram meetings, see Bennett-Levy et al. (2015).

As you will see in a later section on written reflections, an important part of SP/SR involves written reflections about the process that are shared with other group members. While the idea of shared reflections may initially arouse anxieties, the sense of safeness may soon be reinstated once distinctions between private reflections and public reflections, and between reflections on *content* and reflections on *process,* are made. The rule of thumb is that, whereas private personal reflections are likely to include reflections on the content of particular thoughts and uncomfortable feelings, public reflections should involve reflections on the process (e.g., the personal experience of different techniques and implications for therapy with clients) rather than on the content of thoughts or in-depth description of difficult feelings. For instance, you might note uncompassionate thoughts such as "If I can't control my own eating, what right do I have to be a therapist to others?" in a private journal, but in the public domain, it would more appropriate to refer to "thoughts of self-doubt" and an "uncompassionate voice."

The SP/SR Facilitator

A central element in creating a successful SP/SR program and ensuring a sense of safeness is the role of the SP/SR facilitator (Bennett-Levy, Thwaites, Chaddock, & Davis, 2009; Bennett-Levy et al., 2015; Spafford & Haarhoff, 2015). If a group of practitioners are participating in an SP/SR program, then a facilitator or co-facilitators are essential (see Table 4.1 for a quick guide). Depending on the group's familiarity with the SP/SR process, the facilitator's initial role may be to describe the potential benefits of an SP/SR program, which might include directing participants to relevant literature or videos, or having someone describe a personal experience of SP/SR.

TABLE 4.1. A Quick Guide to Facilitating an SP/SR Group

1. Hold a preprogram meeting with the purpose of ensuring that everyone is on the same page, and that there is group input, discussion, and agreement about the structure and process.

2. Either from your own SP/SR experience or from reading the research, explain the value of doing SP/SR.

3. It is particularly important to establish safeness for the group (agreements around confidentiality, personal safeguard strategies, difference between private and public reflections, etc.).

4. Establish agreements around process (e.g., duration of program, choice of modules, timing of meetings, timely postings of reflections).

5. During the SP/SR program, regular reminder e-mails and encouragement are helpful to oil the wheels. Check in with anyone who seems to be "lagging." Inquire if he or she is OK and maybe whether he or she needs anything (e.g., a break for a week).

The facilitator also needs to establish the preconditions for a successful program (e.g., safeness, commitments, contributions, timings) and to "oil the wheels" as the program proceeds. For example, in preprogram meetings, facilitators will work toward establishing group agreements around several pragmatic issues: the length and content of the program, participant commitments (e.g., written reflections), the ground rules for the online discussion forum and/or for face-to-face group meetings, and that all participants have Personal Safeguard Strategies. "Oiling the wheels" of the program once it is under way might include helping participants who are less familiar with online discussion forums to use the technology; reminding group members to post their reflections on the forum by a certain date; encouraging, supporting, and valuing participation; or checking in with a participant if his or her participation seems to have dropped away.

To date, the majority of SP/SR programs (Bennett-Levy et al., 2001; Haarhoff et al., 2011; Spendelow & Butler, 2016), though not all (Bennett-Levy et al., 2003; Davis et al., 2015; Thwaites et al., 2015), have been undertaken with students in university courses. Under these circumstances (or in any situation in which dual relationships may be a concern), in preprogram meetings facilitators need to address any dual relationship issues that might arise from being both a group facilitator and a course teacher. We imagine that formal teaching relationships such as these may be less likely in CFT groups, as at present there are few university-based CFT programs. However, the role of the facilitator is still likely to be crucial in enabling work groups or peer groups to experience maximum benefits. Accordingly, our suggestion is that groups select a facilitator or pair of facilitators that will then take responsibility for the process.

Written Reflections

SP/SR is not just a self-experiential way to learn and refine therapy skills through personal experience of the therapy. The self-reflection part of SP/SR is equally important, as summarized by one SP/SR participant: "Both self-practice and self-reflection were the pivotal components of the course. Without them, it would have been impossible to achieve the level of understanding that comes from applying the material in a meaningful and critical way."

You will find a set of self-reflective questions at the end of each module. Participants consistently report that although writing reflections can be effortful, the benefits are far greater than simply thinking or talking about their experiences. As researchers of reflective writing have found (Bolton, 2010), writing down reflections concretizes our experience and enables us to make sense of it in a way that is rather harder to do by just thinking about it. Furthermore, writing provides a more permanent record of our thinking. We can go back to our writing, reflect on it, add to it, and build upon our understanding. For groups of practitioners undertaking SP/SR, written reflections serve yet another function: They allow group members to learn from one another through sharing reflections, enabling group members to see to what extent their experience of a particular strategy is similar to or different from the experiences of their colleagues.

Written reflections are a core part of the SP/SR process. We strongly recommend that whether you are doing SP/SR individually or in groups, you don't just think about your experience; write it down and reflect on its implications. For further guidance on written reflections in SP/SR, see Bennett-Levy et al. (2015, pp. 20–23) or Haarhoff and Thwaites (2016).

Online Discussion Forums

Most published SP/SR studies have included an online discussion forum. Participants often report that these forums are one of the most valuable parts of the process (Farrand, Perry, & Linsley, 2010; Spafford & Haarhoff, 2015; Thwaites et al., 2015). They can compare their experience of a therapeutic strategy with that of their colleagues. Importantly, also, some SP/SR participants have stronger reflective skills than others. The online discussion forum enables participants to experience the value of the reflective process and to develop their written reflective skills through the modeling of others (Farrand et al., 2010).

As noted previously, creating safeness online is a key requirement. The forum should be open only to members of the training group and the facilitator. At preprogram meetings, participants should decide whether or not postings should be anonymous (different groups tend to vary in this choice); be clear about the difference between private and public reflections (described previously); and develop some ground rules for acceptable and unacceptable postings (e.g., no abuse or criticism). In case there are problems, the facilitator or a nominee should be empowered to enact a moderator role. Some participants may still feel vulnerable (e.g., awareness of being observed by peers and possibly judged). Such feelings should be normalized and recognized as an opportunity for compassion to be extended to oneself and others.

The timetable for posting reflections on discussion forums also needs to be made clear. A forum is of limited value if people are posting randomly about different modules in different weeks, or if people fail to contribute. Groups need to decide when each

SP/SR exercise is to be done, and when written reflections need to be posted; weekly e-mail reminders can help keep reflections on track. When forums are working well, participants not only post reflections about their own experiences, but there is also lively discussion about each other's posts.

Time Management

SP/SR research consistently shows that the single factor that most impedes committed engagement is the perception—and often the reality—of a shortage of time (Haarhoff, Thwaites, & Bennett-Levy, 2015; Spafford & Haarhoff, 2015). Fitting SP/SR into the context of our professional and personal lives takes planning, organization, and commitment. Similarly, in formal teaching programs, if SP/SR is presented as an optional extra, and specific time and course credits are not allocated, then, understandably, participants are less likely to engage with SP/SR programs. Our lives are already busy enough without trying to fit in more around the edges!

For this workbook, we have purposely created short modules that are meant to take no more than 45 minutes on average to complete, apart from those modules that ask you to monitor yourself (e.g., Mindfulness of Self-Criticism Diary, Module 16) or try out new ideas (e.g., Behavioral Experiments in CFT, Module 22) during the week. Our suggestion is to establish an SP/SR routine—a regular time that you set aside to do SP/SR each week.

Preliminary research suggests that if participants short-circuit either the self-practice or the self-reflection component, then the SP/SR effect is diminished (Chaddock, Thwaites, Bennett-Levy, & Freeston, 2014). Those who reflect on both their personal self and therapist self may have better outcomes than those who just reflect on their SP/SR experience from a personal perspective, or those who jump straight to implications for their therapist self without properly experiencing or processing their personal experience (Bennett-Levy & Haarhoff, in press; Chaddock et al., 2014). If you have only a limited number of weeks in which to do CFT SP/SR, we suggest that you select your preferred modules (see the next section), rather than trying to get through them all, but skimming the surface.

Choice of Modules

Ideally you will work through the book systematically, trying out the different practices as you go. However, we realize that this comprehensive approach will not always be practical due to lack of time. You may already be clear about which modules you would most like to do. However, if you are new to CFT (and can't work through the entire book), we would suggest that the following might be considered the core modules, and then you can choose selectively among the remaining modules to round out your experience:

- **Module 1:** Initial Assessment and Identifying a Challenge
- **Module 2:** Three Systems of Emotion
- **Module 3:** Soothing Rhythm Breathing
- **Module 4:** Understanding the Tricky Brain
- **Module 5:** Exploring Old Brain–New Brain Loops
- **Module 6:** Mindful Breathing
- **Module 7:** Shaped by Our Experiences
- **Module 10:** Exploring Attachment Style
- **Module 15:** Unpacking Compassion
- **Module 18:** Different Versions of the Self: The Threat-Based Self
- **Module 19:** Cultivating the Compassionate Self
- **Module 20:** The Compassionate Self in Action
- **Module 24:** Compassion from Self to Others: Skill Building Using Imagery
- **Module 27:** Compassion from Others to Self: Opening to Kindness from Others
- **Module 28:** Compassion Flowing to the Self: Compassionate Letter Writing
- **Module 34:** Maintaining and Enhancing Compassionate Growth

Conclusion

In this chapter, we've reviewed some of the ways in which SP/SR programs can be experienced most effectively. We've emphasized the fundamental importance of creating a sense of safeness, which mirrors the key attributes of CFT. We've also noted how structural aspects of SP/SR—such as recognizing the value of written reflections, managing your time, using online discussion forums well, and being clear about your choice of modules—can enhance your experience. When SP/SR is done in groups, then the role of the facilitator or co-facilitators is of prime importance. In peer groups also, we suggest that a facilitator should be clearly identified, even if this role is shared among group members over time.

As we have seen, SP/SR can be undertaken in a variety of contexts—individually, in co-therapy pairs, groups, supervision, or workshops. There are pros and cons to each of these forms. We suggest weighing these pros and cons, and when you have the opportunity, create a context in which safeness, courage, and self-reflection can flourish.

CHAPTER 5

A Trio of Companions

In writing a book designed to help you learn CFT from the inside out, we want to maximize the experiential aspects of the learning, anchoring your experiences to what the process actually looks and feels like. One way we've chosen to do this is by introducing three therapists and providing examples of their engagement with CFT SP/SR alongside you as you work through the modules. It's our hope that these therapists will model both some of the struggles that CFT can help us address in our lives and clinical work, as well as what it can look like to apply the various processes and practices of CFT to these life challenges.

Your companions in this journey—Fatima, Joe, and Erica—are not real people, at least not as they are presented here. Rather, they represent composites of experiences that we (the authors) have encountered in our own lives and careers, along with experiences reported by our colleagues and supervisees, all adapted for our current purposes. To create a context for understanding the experience of these characters, we spend a bit of time in this chapter giving you a sense of their lives and backgrounds. In doing so, we provide you with some information about them, but leave other details to your imagination—the goal being to maximize readers' ability to relate to the experiences of the characters without getting so specific that we shift the focus from the practices to the nuances of the characters' problems.

Fatima

Fatima is a 28-year-old woman born in the United States to parents who migrated from Pakistan. She is early in her career as a therapist, a career that she has wanted to pursue since her adolescence, when she benefited from seeing a therapist herself after struggling to adjust following the divorce of her parents. Growing up, her relationship with her parents was sometimes unreliable, as her loving but controlling father seemed consumed by his career, and her mother struggled intermittently with depression and alcohol use. When she was 15, Fatima saw a female therapist for about a year, a relationship that she recalls as deeply helpful in assisting her in her schooling and developing friendships over the years. Fatima's network of social support has eroded somewhat recently as she and her peers have found their time increasingly consumed by professional and (in the case of some peers) family commitments. In the moments in which she is most honest with herself, Fatima is aware that although she deeply craves close relationships, she struggles to feel safe in them, and becomes anxious that others will abandon her if she makes mistakes—fears that have prevented her from forming committed relationships with dating partners.

Having always been a hard-working and meticulous student, Fatima excelled in her studies and has recently obtained a position with which she's very pleased: an entry-level therapist position at an adolescent mental health service. Although it doesn't pay quite what she had hoped—enough to afford a modest apartment and her life as a currently single woman, but not much else—she is deeply committed to helping people who struggle, and has a sense of pride in finally becoming a therapist and being able to do so. Her experiences with her first clients were very gratifying for Fatima, as she felt pleased and proud that her clients seemed to appreciate her efforts to help them and seemed to benefit from their contact with her.

Recently, however, Fatima has found herself with a number of very challenging clients. In particular, she has struggled with one of her clients—a volatile female adolescent who, in some ways, reminds her of herself, but whom she feels entirely unable to help. These experiences have triggered a sense of defeat in Fatima and intermittent but powerful experiences of self-doubt in which she questions whether she really "has what it takes" to be a therapist. Having recently attended a training in which the presenter referred to the tendency for therapists to experience shame and self-doubt when faced with such difficult cases, Fatima has decided to build on her CFT skills by addressing her own experiences of shame and self-doubt through CFT SP/SR, which specifically targets such experiences. Having previously benefited from therapy, she has a sense of guarded hopefulness in approaching the program. Fatima also invited her colleague Erica to join her, as they have a casual friendship and are members of the same community peer supervision group.

 Erica

Erica has had a successful career as a therapist for many years and plans to work for another 10 years or so before pursuing retirement. Her current challenge relates to her long-term experience of adapting to her mother's death, occurring 9 months before she decided to begin the SP/SR program. Her mother's death hit Erica hard, deepening occasional feelings of isolation, sadness, and anxiety that she had experienced since divorcing her husband 2 years ago. Erica had a difficult grief process in the 2–3 months after her mother's passing, taking extended time off from work, withdrawing from her social relationships, and attending a number of sessions with a therapist to help her work with the grief.

Although she's largely moved beyond the intense grief she experienced in the first few months following her mother's passing, Erica observes that she has yet to reengage with her previously active social life, and hasn't felt as connected with her clients as she had previously. Since returning to work, she has sometimes felt distracted and as if she is "going through the motions." Previously experiencing herself as a person who is compassionate and warm in both personal and professional relationships, Erica wants to find her way back to experiencing herself in this way. Erica sought out the SP/SR program, thinking it might be a good way to learn CFT, which in turn might help her work with these issues in her own life as well. Erica has been participating in a local peer consultation group with Fatima, and when they learned of their common interest in CFT, the two women decided to go through the Inside Out program together.

 Joe

Joe is a midcareer therapist who has recently changed jobs. This transition worked from a pragmatic standpoint, with the new job being closer to the home he shares with his partner and children and coming with a reasonable increase in pay. However, it has involved a number of new pressures as well. The unit in which he now works is marked by a strong sense of competition among colleagues, with little sense of community or support. His workplace is filled with pressure that seems to flow down from above, with Joe's supervisor driving the therapists to see as many clients as possible and sometimes implying that they could and should be doing more. Joe observes himself having feelings of anger and resentment toward his supervisor, and sometimes finds himself imagining that he would do a better job in his place.

Joe is working hard to succeed in this new position, but he finds himself taking little joy in it. He also feels some frustration that because of the emphasis on productivity, it seems that less of his energy can be devoted to figuring out how to best help his clients. Joe has struggled to find assertive ways to express his needs at work, partially because of the anger and frustration he feels toward his supervisor, and partially due to self-consciousness and not wanting to be seen as the "weak link" or a problem employee. To date, he's coped with all of this by avoiding—trying to "push it down and get on with things"—a strategy that hasn't seemed to help as he observes himself tuning out during meetings and taking his frustration home with him.

Joe has decided that the SP/SR program might help him learn CFT in a way that could help him navigate the challenges at his new job and also help him bring more focus back to his work with his clients.

PART I

Developing Compassionate Understanding

MODULE 1

Initial Assessment
and Identifying a Challenge

As you prepare for the CFT SP/SR program, you might recall the description of the three therapists you met in Chapter 5. We use the challenges in their lives and their experiences as illustrative examples of the different exercises featured in the book.

In this first module, you'll identify a challenge in your own life that can be used as a laboratory for learning how to apply the skills we'll be exploring in the modules to come. This exercise will help you experience what it feels like to apply compassion to a real-life situation. The goal is to set the stage for reflection and exploration around the process of working with this problem, the obstacles that arise when doing so, and how to work with these obstacles—all of which can be valuable in preparing us to apply these strategies with our psychotherapy clients. Related to this exercise, we begin by gathering baseline measures that will give you valuable information to inform your practice and track your progress as you go through the SP/SR program.

✍️ EXERCISE. My Baseline Measures: ECR, FOC, and CEAS-SC

To start with, let's gather some baseline information to help measure the effects of your participation. Just as we often start therapy by collecting some baseline measures of our client's functioning, you'll complete some baseline measures against which you can monitor your progress. We use three measures: an adaptation of the Experiences in Close Relationships (ECR; Fraley, Hefferman, Vicary, & Brumbaugh, 2011) scale designed to get at general experiences of attachment anxiety and avoidance, along with some items selected from Gilbert's Fears of Compassion Scale (FOCS; Gilbert et al., 2011), and the Self-Compassion Engagement and Action subscales of the Compassionate Engagement and Action Scales (CEAS-SC; Gilbert et al., 2017). These measures will help you get a baseline sense of where you are at in relation to these CFT-relevant experiences. Additionally, going through the process may also provide a sense of how clients feel when they're being assessed at the beginning of a course of therapy—and as you would with clients in therapy, we will revisit the measures during the course of the program and then upon completing it. After the measures, you'll write briefly about a current problem or challenge you'd like to work with as you go through the program. In addition to the following measures, you might consider doing a quick Internet search to see if there are any validated measures that more specifically address the challenge or problem you've identified (e.g., anger, self-esteem, social anxiety, worry).

First, let's complete these items adapted from the ECR-RS. To score this form, you'll sum your responses across the first six items to get a measure of attachment avoidance, and then sum the last three items to get a measure of attachment anxiety. You may notice that the direction of the numbers changes in the middle of the measure—we've done this because the first four items are reverse-scored. All you need to do is circle the response that best fits your experience and then sum the numbers you've circled at the end.

ECR-RS: PRETEST

Please read each of the following statements and rate the extent to which you believe each statement best describes your feelings about **close relationships in general.**	Strongly disagree						Strongly agree
1. It helps to turn to people in times of need.	7	6	5	4	3	2	1
2. I usually discuss my problems and concerns with others.	7	6	5	4	3	2	1
3. I usually talk things over with people.	7	6	5	4	3	2	1
4. I find it easy to depend on others.	7	6	5	4	3	2	1
5. I don't feel comfortable opening up to others.	1	2	3	4	5	6	7
6. I prefer not to show others how I feel deep down.	1	2	3	4	5	6	7
7. I often worry that others do not really care about me.	1	2	3	4	5	6	7
8. I'm afraid that other people may abandon me.	1	2	3	4	5	6	7
9. I worry that others won't care about me as much as I care about them.	1	2	3	4	5	6	7

Attachment Avoidance (sum items 1–6): _____

Attachment Anxiety (sum items 7–9): _____

Now take a few minutes to complete and score these items from the FOCS that assess feelings of reluctance to relate compassionately to others, to receive compassion from others, and to direct it toward and receive it from yourself. The items below are just a sampling of a few items from the FOC scale, combined with a few summary items developed for this book (the full, validated scale was too long to include). It hasn't been validated, so please don't use it with clients or in research—you can download the full, validated scale at *https://compassionatemind.co.uk/resources/scales.*

FOCS ITEMS: PRETEST

Please use this scale to rate the extent to which you agree with each statement.	Do not agree at all		Somewhat Agree		Completely Agree
1. Being too compassionate makes people soft and easy to take advantage of.	0	1	2	3	4
2. I fear that being too compassionate makes people an easy target.	0	1	2	3	4
3. I fear that if I am compassionate, some people will become dependent upon me.	0	1	2	3	4
4. I find myself holding back from feeling and expressing compassion toward others.	0	1	2	3	4
5. I try to keep my distance from others even if I know they are kind.	0	1	2	3	4
6. Feelings of kindness from others are somehow frightening.	0	1	2	3	4
7. When people are kind and compassionate toward me, I "put up a barrier."	0	1	2	3	4
8. I have a hard time accepting kindness and caring from others.	0	1	2	3	4
9. I worry that if I start to develop compassion for myself, I will become dependent upon it.	0	1	2	3	4
10. I fear that if I become too compassionate toward myself, I will lose my self-criticism and my flaws will show.	0	1	2	3	4
11. I fear that if I am more self-compassionate, I will become a weak person or my standards will drop.	0	1	2	3	4
12. I struggle with relating kindly and compassionately toward myself.	0	1	2	3	4

Note. This adaptation involves a limited selection of items from the FOC scale as well as additional summary items developed for this book. It was developed so that readers of this book could have a brief way of tracking their progress in working through the modules. As such, this selection of items has not been validated and is not appropriate for use in either research or clinical work. Readers can acquire a copy of the complete, validated version of the scale which is appropriate for research and clinical purposes at *https://compassionatemind.co.uk/resources/scales.*

Fears of Extending Compassion (sum items 1–4):	_____
Fears of Receiving Compassion (sum items 5–8):	_____
Fears of Self-Compassion (sum items 9–12):	_____

Now for a final brief measure, the self-compassion engagement and action subscales from the CEAS-SC

CEAS-SC: PRETEST

When I'm distressed or upset by things . . .	Never									Always
1. I am *motivated* to engage and work with my distress when it arises.	1	2	3	4	5	6	7	8	9	10
2. I *notice* and am *sensitive* to my distressed feelings when they arise in me.	1	2	3	4	5	6	7	8	9	10
3. I am *emotionally moved* by my distressed feelings or situations.	1	2	3	4	5	6	7	8	9	10
4. I *tolerate* the various feelings that are part of my distress.	1	2	3	4	5	6	7	8	9	10
5. I *reflect on* and *make sense* of my feelings of distress.	1	2	3	4	5	6	7	8	9	10
6. I am *accepting, noncritical,* and *non-judgmental* of my feelings of distress.	1	2	3	4	5	6	7	8	9	10
7. I direct my *attention* to what is likely to be helpful to me.	1	2	3	4	5	6	7	8	9	10
8. I *think* about and come up with helpful ways to cope with my distress.	1	2	3	4	5	6	7	8	9	10
9. I take the *actions* and do the things that will be helpful to me.	1	2	3	4	5	6	7	8	9	10
10. I create inner feelings of *support, helpfulness,* and *encouragement*.	1	2	3	4	5	6	7	8	9	10

| Compassionate Engagement (sum items 1–6): | _____ |
| Compassionate Action (sum items 7–10): | _____ |

Just as with clients, you'll have a chance to repeat these measures at the mid- and end points of the program so that you can see the progress you've made. Now that you have completed the baseline assessment, let's identify a challenge or problem that you can use as a reference point as you learn about CFT from the inside out.

 EXERCISE. Identifying My Challenge or Problem

We all face a variety of challenging situations and problems in our lives. As mental health professionals, sometimes these problems occur in the clinic or therapy room, and even when they initially occur outside of the professional context, sometimes they find their way into our professional lives. In this exercise, you'll identify a challenge or problem in your professional and/or personal life that you'll then be able to use as a point of reference as you work through the remainder of the book.

To begin, we recommend that you set aside some time to do the exercise in a quiet, comfortable place where you'll be undisturbed. Then take some time to reflect on your experience of yourself as a therapist (or on your personal life). Reflect on the difficult feelings that sometimes arise for you, and consider the situations or experiences you face that tend to trigger you or "push your buttons." Perhaps these are situations in which you find yourself responding in ways you aren't comfortable with, or which don't reflect the sort of person you wish to be. Or perhaps they are situations in which you feel trapped or unsure of what to do, or which prompt experiences of self-doubt, self-criticism, or shame in you.

If you're focusing on your "therapist self," these might involve struggles with particular clients, types of clients, supervisors, supervisees, or colleagues. Are there situations in your work life that you find yourself dreading, avoiding, or ruminating about? It could be frustration about not making progress with a particular client, or not getting what you need from a supervisor. It could be stress related to productivity expectations in the workplace, or feelings of anger when clients no-show at the last minute or cancel without calling. Or you may have feelings of insecurity or dread around working with certain clients or even colleagues.

 EXAMPLE: Fatima's Challenging Problem

Fatima identified a particular client with whom she is struggling, who both reminds her of herself at a younger age and who is directing hostility toward Fatima. This hostile response has prompted feelings of self-doubt around her competency as a therapist, and feelings of wanting to avoid meeting with the client.

EXAMPLE: Joe's Challenging Problem

Having recently changed jobs, Joe now finds himself in a position with high productivity expectations, and with a supervisor he experiences as overbearing and more concerned with the number of clients seen than with the quality of care being provided. Joe has been experiencing feelings of irritability and anger around these areas, and is troubled that these feelings have "seeped out" into his personal life in the form of sometimes snapping at his wife and children.

You may find that the problem you'd like to work with occurs more in your personal life. Such problems may be restricted to your personal life, or they may also find their way into your professional life, as we see in Erica's example.

 EXAMPLE: Erica's Challenging Problem

Erica's choice to begin the SP/SR program was preceded by a challenging 6-month period following the death of her mother. For the first couple of months following her mother's death, Erica struggled with overwhelming grief, taking an extended time off from work, and pulling back from social activities. Although her grief has softened over time, Erica has struggled to reengage with her life, and she hasn't really resumed the activities that fell away during her period of intense grief. Most troublingly, despite previously feeling very passionate about her work, she's observed that her motivation has yet to return, and has noticed herself fantasizing about retirement and experiencing self-criticism around not feeling as engaged and committed to her clients as she's used to being.

In the following box, make a list of any challenges or problems you currently face.

CHALLENGING PROBLEMS

Reviewing the challenging problems you've just identified, consider which you would like to focus on as you work through the modules. Select a problem that activates threat emotions such as fear, anger, or anxiety at a moderate level of intensity (typically 40–75% on a 0–100 scale of distress), but not an extreme level (e.g., no higher than 75%). Because CFT was developed particularly to help people who struggle with shame and self-criticism, it would be a particularly good fit to select a problem that triggers aspects of these experiences. Finally, as we discussed in Chapter 3, we strongly recommend that you *not* choose a problem that is too intense—which causes you a level of distress that, in your judgment, would cause you to make a recommendation for treatment, were you to see it in another person. In this way, it is probably good to avoid selecting situations such as unresolved trauma, major relationship problems, or other situations that would cause you significant distress if not resolved by the end of the SP/SR program.

Once you've selected your challenge or problem, describe it in the following box. It doesn't have to be a lengthy description; provide as much detail as will be helpful to clarify the issue in your mind, for current and future reference.

MY CHALLENGING PROBLEMS

Now that you've completed the measures and identified your challenging problem, it will be helpful to reflect on the experience—a critical part of SP/SR that we repeat throughout the book.

Self-Reflective Questions

Consider your experience of the exercises in this module. Did you find doing the measures easy, difficult, or uncomfortable? What was it about the experience, and your reaction, that made it so?

_____

_____

_____

_____

_____

_____

_____

_____

_____

_____

_____

_____

_____

_____

How was it to identify the challenging problem? What motivations, emotions, thoughts, or bodily sensations did you notice as you went through the exercise? How do you understand or make sense of those experiences?

_____

_____

_____

_____

_____

_____

_____

_____

_____

_____

_____

_____

_____

Reflecting on the experience of identifying your problem and completing the initial measures, does anything stand out that might inform how you approach this process with your clients? How might using SP/SR to go through this process yourself affect how you approach the initial assessment and problem clarification process with your clients?

_____

_____

_____

_____

_____

_____

_____

_____

_____

_____

_____

_____

_____

What have you taken away from this module that might be worth continuing to reflect on over the next week or so?

_____

_____

_____

_____

_____

_____

_____

_____

_____

_____

_____

_____

Three Systems of Emotion

In the previous module, you completed some initial assessment measures and identified a specific challenging situation or problem. In doing so, we prompted you to identify a problem that stirred up some uncomfortable emotions, such as anger, anxiety, or frustration. A primary aspect of CFT involves helping our clients make realizations that set the stage for the arising of compassion for themselves and others. An example of such a realization is that when we take a close look at our evolved brains, our emotions, and how they work, we learn that there are numerous factors that powerfully shape our experience and set us up for struggle—factors that we didn't create or design and which aren't our fault (Gilbert, 2009, 2010). In this module, we explore how CFT contextualizes emotions in ways that are designed to help clients move from criticizing and attacking themselves to a compassionate perspective that understands these experiences as unchosen products of how our evolved brains work.

A foundational piece of this is the three-circles model of emotions, introduced in Chapter 2, which organizes human emotions and motives into three systems (see Figure M2.1). These systems are anchored to evolved functions that help us (1) detect and respond to things we perceive as threats (the threat system); (2) identify, pursue, and experience reward for achieving goals (the drive and resource acquisition system); and (3) experience feelings of safeness, peacefulness, calm, and connection (the soothing and safeness system).

Reflecting on the Three Systems

For the exercise that follows, start by pausing to think about how you're feeling now and how you've felt over the past week. Considering your experiences of threat, drive, and safeness during this time, draw the relative size of your three systems, thinking about how much these emotional experiences have tended to "show up" in your life lately.

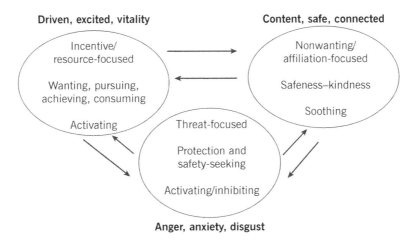

FIGURE M2.1. Three systems of emotion regulation. From Gilbert (2009), *The Compassionate Mind*. Reprinted with permission from Little, Brown Book Group.

You'll then be prompted to explore experiences that might be related to these patterns of activation—thoughts and feelings you may have had, as well as how these relate to things that have happened in your life, perhaps particularly in relation to the problem you identified in Module 1. Finally, you'll consider how the three systems might be interacting to shape your emotional reality, and you'll reflect on your experience of the exercise.

 EXAMPLE: Fatima's Reflection

Fatima drew her three systems, with the size of each circle indicating how strongly experiences of threat, drive, and safeness colored her recent experience of life.

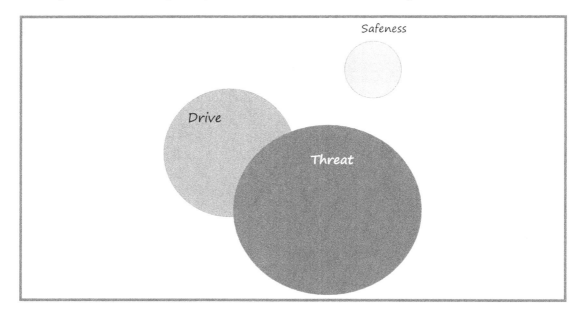

What reflections do you have on your drawing of the three systems?
*Well, it's pretty clear that my recent experience has mostly been one of threat. My threat circle is much larger than the others. My drive circle is still pretty big because I really **want** to be a good therapist and to help my clients, but it's partially blocked and covered up by the threat. I haven't felt as safe lately, so my safeness circle is smaller.*

How does your drawing reflect your recent life experience?
Recently I've been experiencing more threat. I've been doubting my ability to be a good therapist, anxious about the fact that I don't seem to have been able to help Alex, my client, and frustrated with myself about that. It gets in the way of my drive to help people and really make a difference, and it's hard to feel motivated to work with my clients when I'm frequently doubting myself. Although I have moments of safeness with my supervisor, I don't know that she really understands how much this has shaken me.

Do you notice any interactions between your three systems?
Definitely. The threat is definitely blocking my drive to succeed. Instead of being excited to go to work, I sometimes dread it. The whole thing—seeing clients, writing progress notes, even things like answering e-mails—has seemed like more of a chore, and I've found myself avoiding it and distracting myself by zoning out or playing games on my phone.

What did you learn from this exercise that you'd like to remember?
How this feeling of struggling with my client hasn't just made me feel threatened, but that it's also really impacted my motivation around being a therapist. I used to love this work, but this threat seems to have blocked some of that. It also makes me think I need to talk with my supervisor to help her understand how much this has affected me, so that maybe she can help me feel safer at work.

Now, complete the exercise for yourself. Take a few moments to reflect upon how you feel now and how you have felt generally in the past week or two. Try to find some time to pause and reflect on your three systems, perhaps during a few quiet moments or a walk. You might want to use colored pencils or markers (in CFT, we use red to indicate threat, blue for drive, and green for safeness). Draw the circles to relative scale, indicating how large each emotion system is in relation to the others.

 EXERCISE. Reflecting on My Three Systems

In the following box, draw your three systems, with the size of each circle indicating how strongly experiences of threat (fear, anxiety, anger), drive (excitement, interest), and safeness (calm, peaceful, content) color your recent experience of life.

What reflections do you have on your drawing of the three systems?

How does your drawing reflect your recent life experience?

Do you notice any interactions between your three systems?

What did you learn from this exercise that you'd like to remember?

Checking In with the Three Circles

In Modules 6 and 14, we explore mindfulness, which involves learning to relate to our experiences in present-focused, accepting, and non-judgmental ways. This way of considering our experiences sets the stage for compassion and self-compassion to emerge, particularly when we learn to direct this mindful awareness toward our own thoughts and emotions (as opposed to, say, relating to these experiences with judgment and criticism). However, we can get a jump-start on this mindful awareness by "checking in" with our three circles. In doing this, we'll briefly reflect on the three circles and try to notice and rate how much we feel threatened, driven, and safe in the current moment. Try just to notice these experiences without judging them—just notice that "this is what my experience is like right now." Checking in can help us get in the habit of noticing the activation of these experiences in ourselves. It can also help us recognize that a lot of the time, we aren't just feeling one thing; we can see patterns of relative activation across the "circles." Finally, if we notice we're out of balance when we check in with the three systems, we may decide to do something about that. For example, if we notice that we're feeling quite threatened, we might engage in some soothing rhythm breathing (introduced in the Module 3) to slow things down and get our safeness system "online."

EXERCISE. Checking In with the Three Circles

Take a moment to bring your attention to the emotions and motivations you find yourself experiencing right now. Consider: "How threatened do I feel right now? Do I notice feelings of anger, fear, anxiety, apprehension, or disgust?" Then try to notice how driven you feel: "Do I notice feelings of desire, excitement, or the motivation to pursue a goal?" Finally, try to notice how safe you feel: "Am I experiencing feelings of peacefulness, calm, safeness, and contentment?" See if you can rate these sensations on the following scale:

How threatened do I feel right now?

1	2	3	4	5	6	7	8	9	10

Not at all threatened   Moderately threatened   Very threatened

How driven do I feel right now?

1	2	3	4	5	6	7	8	9	10

Not at all driven   Moderately driven   Very driven

How safe, content, and at ease do I feel right now?

1	2	3	4	5	6	7	8	9	10

Not at all safe   Moderately safe   Very safe

 Self-Reflective Questions

What was it like using the three systems diagram to understand your experience? How much did it ring true?

_____

_____

_____

_____

_____

_____

_____

_____

_____

_____

_____

_____

_____

_____

How did you know which system you were in? What kinds of differences did you notice in your experience of threat, drive, and safeness? What differences did you notice in how the systems organized you bodily experience? Your thoughts? Your emotions? Your motivations?

_____

_____

_____

_____

_____

_____

_____

_____

_____

_____

_____

_____

_____

Did any blocks, distress, or discomfort arise? If so, how do you make sense of that?

_____

_____

_____

_____

_____

_____

_____

_____

_____

_____

What initial ideas do you have about how you might use the three systems with your clients?

_____

_____

_____

_____

_____

_____

_____

_____

_____

_____

_____

MODULE 3

Soothing Rhythm Breathing

When activated, our threat system's influence can direct our physiology, emotions, attention, thinking, and behavior in ways that can cause us problems. However, the soothing and safeness system—underpinned by the parasympathetic nervous system—evolved to play an important role in helping regulate threat system activation in humans. In this module, we explore how we can practice a way of working with the physiology of our soothing system to help bring balance to things after the threat system has been activated.

A growing body of research links learning how to work with the breath, and in particular, slowing down the breath and working with its smoothness and rhythm, with activation of the parasympathetic "brake" system that helps slow down heart rate, lower blood pressure, and is associated with happiness and resilience (Berntson, Cacioppo, & Quigley, 1993; Pal & Velkumary, 2004; Brown & Gerbarg, 2005; Kaushik, Kaushik, Mahajan, & Rajesh, 2006; Kok & Frederickson, 2010; Jerath, Edry, Barnes, & Jerath, 2006; Porges, Doussard-Roosevelt, & Maiti, 1994). With practice, learning to work with the breath can be a powerful way of engaging with threat emotions by stimulating physiological processes that are helpful in balancing threat-based arousal. Although soothing rhythm breathing may not completely dissipate threat emotions, it can soften them and help us shift into a more mindful, intentional perspective as we slow things down and gain a bit of distance between our awareness and the urgency of our threat-focused emotions. Soothing rhythm breathing can also create some space that our new brains can use to reconnect with our compassionate intentions, recognize that we're struggling, validate our own experience, and consider things from a broader perspective through questions such as "If I were at my best—my kindest, wisest, most courageous, and most compassionate—how would I want to handle this situation?"

EXERCISE. Soothing Rhythm Breathing

For this exercise, find a quiet, comfortable place where you can practice without interruption for at least 5–10 minutes. With practice, you'll be able to use soothing rhythm breathing in any number of situations and settings, but to start, it helps to have a comfortable, relatively soothing environment—or at least one that isn't too chaotic.

Sit comfortably in an upright position with chest open, feet flat on the floor, hands gently settled on your lap, and holding your head in an upright, comfortable, and alert position. Feel free to allow your eyes to close or to keep them open, as you prefer. If you keep them open, you may wish to allow your gaze to drop to the floor 6–8 feet in front of you (while continuing to hold your head in an upright position) and "soften" your gaze (unfocusing a bit). The key is to hold your body in a comfortable position with an open and upright posture (you don't want to slump or slouch such that your body folds in on itself).

Breathing in and out through your nose, start by gently bringing a soothing rhythm to your breathing—a rhythm that feels comfortable to your body. After 30 seconds or so, begin to see what it feels to imagine that, as you breathe out, you feel your body slowing down a little. Or maybe as you breathe out, you just notice that your legs are resting on the chair and your feet are on the floor.

Now, begin to allow your breath to slow to a rate of 4–5 seconds on the inbreath, holding for a moment, and then another 4–5 seconds on the outbreath. We're looking for a rate of 6 or so breaths per minute. Breathe down into your abdomen, deeply enough that it's comfortable (you feel like you're getting plenty of air).

Breathe like this for 2 minutes or so, bringing your attention to the sense of slowing in the body . . . slowing down the body, slowing down the mind. Feel free to take more time if you'd like.

As you complete the exercise, allow yourself to notice how focusing on slowing the breath has impacted your body and mind.

Upon finishing this exercise (and all CFT exercises), it's useful to consider the experience, noticing what was helpful as well as any obstacles that may have arisen during the process.

What did you notice during the soothing rhythm breathing exercise?

How did it impact your mental state? Did you notice any shifts in your body, your emotions, or your thinking?

How did you feel about the exercise? Did you enjoy it? If so, what did you enjoy? If you didn't enjoy it, what didn't you enjoy about it?

Were there any obstacles that got in the way?

If there were obstacles, how might you work with them so that the exercise might be more helpful for you?

It's important to recognize that not every practice will be helpful for everyone, or will have the same function for everyone. Some clients (e.g., clients with a history of physical trauma such as sexual assault) can find focusing on bodily sensations such as the breath to be very aversive. For these clients, focusing on the breath can function more like an exposure trial than as a way of activating the safeness system. If the process that you're trying to target is soothing and slowing down the body, it would probably be better to find another practice (or to work collaboratively with your client to find another practice) that you experience as soothing. For example:

- Focusing on a tactile sensation, such as holding something soft like a pillow or stuffed animal, a smooth stone, or anything else you find soothing.
- Listening to a soothing piece of music or other sound, such as ocean waves or the wind through trees (such sounds can easily be found for free on the Internet in sites such as YouTube).
- Gently petting an animal.
- Focusing attention on any other sensory experience that you find soothing.

The idea is to find a sensory experience that can help slow the body and mind, giving us the opportunity to shift into a more soothing, compassionate frame of mind.

As with almost any practice, the effects of soothing rhythm breathing increase as it is practiced over time and across situations. Initially, it's best to practice when you are already relatively calm, and then gradually begin to use it in situations that increasingly trigger the threat system. One common obstacle to this straightforward practice for both therapists and clients is simply forgetting to practice, so take a moment to consider when you might practice, and how you might remind yourself so that you don't forget.

PRACTICE PLAN

What times of day would be good for me to practice soothing rhythm breathing?

What might help me remember to practice so that I can do so consistently?

Self-Reflective Questions

Did you enjoy learning about soothing rhythm breathing—or not? Did any obstacles come up for you? If so, what were they?

_____

_____

_____

_____

_____

_____

_____

_____

_____

_____

_____

_____

_____

Considering your practice plan to use soothing rhythm breathing in your daily life, what obstacles do you anticipate might get in the way? How might you work with them to help make your practice plan a success?

_____

_____

_____

_____

_____

_____

_____

_____

_____

_____

_____

_____

_____

_____

Reflecting on your own experiences of soothing rhythm breathing, what problems do you anticipate may arise in working with clients? Can you think of any clients for whom this practice might be helpful? What would make it so? What about clients for whom it might be too much of a challenge? How might you know?

_____

_____

_____

_____

_____

_____

_____

_____

_____

_____

_____

_____

_____

_____

Based on your experience, how do you think soothing rhythm breathing might be related to the successful cultivation of compassion for yourself and/or others?

_____

_____

_____

_____

_____

_____

_____

_____

_____

_____

_____

_____

_____

_____

Understanding the Tricky Brain

A fundamental idea in CFT is that *human beings inherit brains and bodies that were shaped by evolution to operate in ways that we didn't choose or design, and which aren't our fault.* This realization is core to CFT—that many of the experiences that cause the most distress for us and for our clients are nobody's fault. Rather, they are a result of the ways that our brains and bodies—and through them, our experience of emotions—were shaped by evolution (Gilbert, 2009, 2010, 2014). This module and the next explore this theme further by focusing on "old-brain" processes and "new-brain" processes and how these can interact.

Old-Brain Emotions and Motives

Different parts of our brains—and the functions for which they are responsible—evolved at different times. We have ancient structures in our brains that trigger many of the same powerful emotions, motives, and behaviors in us as were experienced by our reptilian and mammalian ancestors (Panksepp & Biven, 2012). For example, like these ancestors, humans experience powerful emotional states such as fear, anger, and lust, coupled with equally powerful motives focused on aggression, avoiding pain, and mating.

In considering these emotions, it can be useful to also notice the experiences that tend to trigger their arising. Emotional reactions can be triggered by external events and situations as well as by internal experiences such as thoughts, memories, and even physical sensations. Let's take a few moments to consider an old-brain emotion and how it can play out.

Exploring Old-Brain Threat Responses

 EXAMPLE: Fatima's Reflection

Choose an example of an old-brain threat emotion with which you sometimes struggle:

Fear, definitely fear. And anxiety, but that's related to the fear.

What situations tend to trigger this emotion?

When my client ridicules my attempts to be helpful. She seems to delight in letting me know that nothing I do is helping her, and it seems like she's right. It's gotten so that even thinking about her makes me fearful.

What is it like as the emotion arises? For example, is your experience one of *choosing* to feel this emotion, or does it just arise within you—and what is that like?

It just comes up in me, and once it's there, it's completely stifling—almost like being choked. I feel like I'm filled with fear, just frozen with it.

What motivations come along with this emotion? What do you find yourself wanting to do?

Avoid. I've found myself hoping that she'll cancel sessions, and I've put off writing progress notes. I even called in sick once when I wasn't really ill, because I just wasn't up to dealing with her on that day.

What behaviors do you engage in as you experience this emotion? What do you find yourself doing?

Like I wrote above, it's more what I find myself not doing. I delay writing progress notes and even though she's one of my more challenging clients, I don't do as much work outside of the session to prepare for our interaction as I would normally do. It's hard to bring myself to focus on her for any length of time.

Now consider a threat emotion you've experienced lately. Try to notice the different aspects of this feeling—when and how it comes up in you, and how it shapes your attention. Observe the motivation the emotion carries with it: What do you find yourself wanting to do when this experience arises in you? Finally, what do you find yourself doing—how does your motivation translate into behavior?

EXERCISE. Exploring My Old-Brain Threat Responses

Choose an example of an old-brain threat emotion with which you sometimes struggle:

What situations tend to trigger this emotion?

What is it like as the emotion arises? For example, is your experience one of *choosing* to feel this emotion, or does it just arise within you—and what is that like?

What motivations come along with this emotion? What do you find yourself wanting to do?

What behaviors do you engage in as you experience this motivation? What do you find yourself doing?

New-Brain Thinking, Imagery, and Meaning Making

Although we humans share many powerful old-brain emotions, motives, and behaviors with our nonhuman ancestors, unlike these ancestors, we also have fancy "new-brain" capacities as well: We can engage in symbolic thought, create detailed fantasies and mental imagery, assign meaning to our experiences, and engage in mental time travel that allows us to plan and reminisce. This capacity for higher-order thought brings with it a host of unique problems: We can ruminate on our struggles; reflect on what our experiences, motives, and behaviors *mean about us*; and interpret and experience almost any thought or perception we have in an almost infinite number of ways, depending upon the physical and mental contexts in which these experiences are framed (Villatte, Villatte, & Hayes, 2016).

CFT emphasizes the importance of recognizing these brain capacities as part of the fundamental challenge of being human. Using a simplified language designed for ease of understanding, we can recognize that old-brain emotions can act very powerfully to shape both the content (what we focus on, think about, and imagine) and process (whether our thinking and attention are narrow or broad, reflective or filled with urgency) of our new-brain capacities for thought, imagery, and meaning making. Let's take a look at how this process can play out.

Reflecting on New-Brain Thoughts, Imagery, and Meaning Making

In this brief exercise, we continue with the threat emotion you identified in the previous exercise and explore what is going on in the new brain when this threat emotion comes up. First, let's consider Fatima's reflection.

 EXAMPLE: Fatima's Reflection

> **Using the threat emotion you identified above, consider the thoughts and mental images that tend to arise when you are feeling like that.**
>
> **What thoughts come up?** *I just keep ruminating on my fears of not being able to help her, and about the idea that I might not be cut out to be a therapist. Thoughts like "I can't do this." "I just don't have what it takes." "She sees through me." "I'm a fraud."*
>
> **Are there any mental images or fantasies that accompany the emotion? What are they like?** *I keep playing the situation in my mind over and over again—my client telling me that I'm not helping her, watching her struggle, and not being able to do anything about it. I also picture my supervisor in my mind, telling me that maybe I'm not cut out to be a therapist after all, although she's never actually said anything like that.*

> **Considering the emotion and the situation that prompted it, what meaning do you assign to it? What does it mean about you or your life that you had this experience?** *I guess I feel like it means I don't have what it takes. Therapists are supposed to know what they're doing, and I obviously don't. I should be confident, and I'm clearly not. It's like I'm worried that I'm this child playing at something that she has no business at, and that I need to wake up and face the real world.*

Considering Fatima's example, take a few minutes to reflect on what it's like for you when that old-brain threat emotion comes up, and the thoughts and imagery that arise along with them. Consider both the content and the quality with which these experiences play out (e.g., ruminatively thinking the same thought or playing out the same scene again and again in your mind).

 EXERCISE. Exploring My New-Brain Thoughts, Imagery, and Meaning Making

> **Using the threat emotion you identified above, consider the thoughts and mental images that tend to arise when you are feeling like that.**
>
> **What thoughts come up?**
>
>
>
>
>
>
>
>
>
> **Are there any mental images or fantasies that accompany the emotion? What are they like?**

Considering the emotion and the situation that prompted it, what meaning do you assign to it? What does it mean about you or your life that you had this experience?

Self-Reflective Questions

How easy or difficult was it to observe old-brain processes? How easy or difficult was it to observe new-brain processes? What made it so?

_____

_____

_____

_____

_____

_____

_____

_____

_____

_____

_____

_____

_____

Did you notice any compassion (or reluctance to experience compassion) arising as you focused on these experiences stemming from your old brain and new brain? How do you understand the relationship between compassion—or the absence of compassion—and these threat emotions? What sense do you make of this?

_____

_____

_____

_____

_____

_____

_____

_____

_____

_____

_____

_____

_____

Reflecting on this experience of threat emotions as they manifested in old and new brains, does anything stand out that might inform how you engage clients with these processes?

_____

_____

_____

_____

_____

_____

_____

_____

_____

_____

_____

_____

_____

_____

How does your experience of this module relate to your understanding of the CFT model?

_____

_____

_____

_____

_____

_____

_____

_____

_____

_____

_____

_____

_____

Exploring Old Brain–New Brain Loops

In CFT, as we consider the functioning of our emotional old brains and our thinking new brains that we explored in the previous module, it's important to also observe that these different aspects of mental experience can interact to form "loops" that can serve to maintain tricky emotional states (Gilbert, 2010; Kolts, 2016). These interactions are depicted in Figure M5.1.

Let's consider how these loops can work by revisiting the experience of a couple of our compassionate companions.

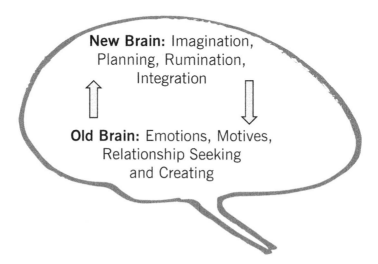

FIGURE M5.1. Old brain–new brain loops. From Gilbert (2009). *The Compassionate Mind.* Reprinted with permission from Little, Brown Book Group.

EXAMPLE: Fatima's Reflection

Let's consider the ways your old brain and new brain can form loops in response to a challenging experience.

First, briefly describe a challenging situation.

A couple of weeks ago my client actually told me, "I don't even know why I come here. I don't think you can help me."

What old-brain emotions and motivations were triggered by the situation? What was happening in your body?

I was terrified, but also angry. I didn't know whether to run out of the room or to say, "Well, you little shit, if you would try participating in the therapy, it might help!" But mostly I was scared that she was right. My heart was racing, and I felt like I was breathing so hard that she must be able to notice. I also got dry mouth, and I felt really cold, even after I put on my sweater.

What thoughts and imagery played out for you?

Aside from what I wrote above, I kept thinking that she was probably right—that I don't know how to help her, and that even her resisting participating in the therapy was my fault because I obviously don't know how to motivate her. I just kept thinking, "I don't know what to do!" I was also imagining her storming out and my peers learning of my failure with her . . . that sort of thing. It stuck with me for a long time after the session was over.

Now consider how these different aspects of your experience may have interacted to form loops. How might they have influenced one another? For example, how did your feelings impact your attention and what you thought and imagined? How did your thoughts and imagery impact your feelings?

After she said that and I responded—I don't even remember what I said—she went on to talk about some things she had coming up this week. But I have no idea what she was talking about. I was lost in the anxiety, just thinking about how I was a failure and that I didn't know how to help her. My heart was racing and I just couldn't calm down, and I kept wondering if she could tell. It impacted me for the next several hours as I kept replaying what she said in my mind: "I don't even know why I come here." It was like it was happening over and over again, and I know it kept me caught in the anxiety. I was so unsettled that I skipped lunch—my stomach was uneasy and I'd completely lost my appetite, just feeling upset.

Now let's take a moment to catch up with Joe, who's been struggling with anger related to a situation with his supervisor and his demands at work.

EXAMPLE: Joe's Reflection

Let's consider the ways your old brain and new brain can form loops in response to a challenging experience.

First, briefly describe a challenging situation.

I went to a staffing meeting last week, where we're supposed to discuss new cases and give progress updates on the clients we've been working with. I have a case that I wanted some input on because it's really complicated and I don't quite have a handle on things yet. Well, Gary [Joe's supervisor] comes in late after we've already started, and interrupts things to go on the same monologue about productivity that he gives us constantly. It's always the same thing: We need to see more clients, provide more documentation, blah, blah, blah. He took up the whole time, and we never did get to talk about our cases. It's not helpful, either. Susan asked him a direct question about how to handle no-shows, and he talked for another 20 minutes without ever answering her question.

What old-brain emotions and motivations were triggered by the situation? What was happening in your body?

I was furious. I didn't say anything, just fumed for the rest of the afternoon. It just feels like banging your head against the wall. I felt like a white-hot ball of energy, like I was going to explode. When I got back to my office, I just sat there with my jaw clenched, all tense and seething.

What thoughts and imagery played out for you?

I just kept thinking what a waste of time it was, and wondering how he even has a job. Lots of negativity about the job, too. Things like "I hate this. This job sucks. I can't take this anymore." I imagined getting up and yelling at him, storming out of the room. Of course, I didn't do anything. I just sat there and took it.

Now consider how these different aspects of your experience may have interacted to form loops. How might they have influenced one another? For example, how did your feelings impact your attention and what you thought and imagined? How did your thoughts and imagery impact your feelings?

Looking back, it seems clear that it all fed back on itself. I was thinking and imagining all that angry stuff, which just kept me angry, and which definitely showed up in my body as well. I was focused so sharply on what had happened and how angry I was that I didn't get much work done the rest of the afternoon—I had a mound of paperwork and had a hard time focusing on any of it. After a while I even got frustrated with myself, seeing myself just sitting there seething like that. I felt really ashamed. That's not the guy I want to be.

Now try the exercise yourself. See if you can bring up a recent experience in which your threat system was activated. Once again, begin by exploring your old-brain emotions and motives and your then new-brain thoughts and imagery, this time in terms of how you found yourself responding to this situation. Then consider how these different aspects of your experience may have interacted to shape the way those emotions played out in you in an ongoing fashion.

EXERCISE. Exploring My Old Brain–New Brain Loops

Let's consider the ways your old brain and new brain can form loops in response to a challenging experience.

First, briefly describe a challenging situation.

What old-brain emotions and motivations were triggered by the situation? What was happening in your body?

What thoughts and imagery played out for you?

Now consider how these different aspects of your experience may have interacted to form loops. How might they have influenced one another? For example, how did your feelings impact your attention and what you thought and imagined? How did your thoughts and imagery impact your feelings?

Self-Reflective Questions

What sense did you have of the idea of loops through your self-practice experience? Was this looping something you were able to experience directly?

As you reflect on your experience of how the old brain and new brain can interact in tricky ways, does anything stand out that might be useful with your clients? Can you think of any clients for whom this exploration might be helpful? How might you use it with them?

_____

_____

_____

_____

_____

_____

_____

_____

_____

_____

_____

_____

_____

MODULE 6

Mindful Breathing

In modern secular health care, the practice of mindfulness has been systematized into effective therapeutic programs, for example, in the treatment of recurrent depression (Segal, Williams, & Teasdale, 2012) and the management of chronic medical conditions and pain (Kabat-Zinn, 2013). Mindfulness is also important to CFT: it helps us develop an awareness of our mental experiences as they occur (as thoughts, feelings, and sensations) rather than getting caught up in them, and it helps us become more familiar with how our minds work. If we're going to bring compassion to difficult experiences, we first need to be *aware* of them. This module introduces mindful breathing as an example of how mindfulness is integrated into CFT.

Mindful Breathing

In mindful breathing, we give ourselves the attentional anchor of the breath and the sensations it creates in the body. The task is simple, but not easy: As the mind becomes distracted and moves away from the intended focus of the practice, we note where the mind has wandered to and gently return our attention to the breath in the body. The aim of the practice isn't to create a "blank" mind, but rather to deal with mind-wandering in a skillful and non-judgmental manner. The distractions aren't a problem or mistake; rather, they provide an opportunity to train our attention by helping us learn to notice movement in the mind. They can also be a cue for offering compassion to ourselves as we realize how wildly and unpredictably our minds can jump about—our minds can be very tricky!

Before you begin your practice, find a quiet place where you are unlikely to be disturbed. It is best to undertake the practice sitting on a chair, rather than lying down, as the intention is to be awake and alert. If you are guiding yourself via the written instructions that follow, it can be helpful to set a timer, perhaps for 10 minutes, to remind you when to finish the exercise.

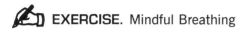 **EXERCISE.** Mindful Breathing

1. Sit in a posture that is relaxed but upright and alert.

2. Close your eyes or lower and soften the focus of your gaze.

3. Bring awareness to your bodily sensations. You might begin by focusing on the contact points of your body with the outside world (e.g., your feet as they connect with the floor). Widen your attention to take in the whole of the body, allowing the sensations you notice to be just as they are. Explore what it feels like to let go of wanting things to be a certain way.

4. Bring attention to your breath wherever you notice it most strongly in your body. This might be in your abdomen as the breath moves your stomach muscles in and out; it might be at tip of your nose where the breath enters and leaves the body; or it might be in any other area that you choose. Follow each breath with your attention, noticing the changing physical sensations of the inbreath and the outbreath, and the pauses between them.

5. Breathe at a rate and rhythm that feels natural and comfortable to you. There is no need to control your breathing in any way.

6. Continue to rest your attention on the breath. When your mind wanders to thoughts, images, other sensations or emotions, gently bring your attention back to the breath. Each time you notice that your attention has wandered from the breath, realize that this is a moment of mindfulness: a "waking up" to the movement of your mind. It also provides an opportunity to bring compassion to your mind and your experiences, as you return your attention to your breathing with kindness and patience.

7. Continue with the practice for 10 minutes, or for however long you feel comfortable. As you finish the exercise, gently bring your attention back to your external environment, taking time to readjust.

To really reap the benefits of mindfulness practice, you might choose to practice the exercise on a daily basis, writing down your observations after each practice. It can be helpful to aim to practice for 5 days out of every 7. Here's an example of Erica's record of her mindful breathing:

 EXAMPLE: Erica's Mindful Breathing Record

Day and time of practice	Duration	What I noticed
Monday 6:00 P.M.	5 min	I noticed my mind wandering, but I went with it and kept bringing my attention back to my breathing.
Tuesday 6:15 P.M.	10 min	I focused on my breath in my tummy and found it easier to stay with the exercise. I noticed my body becoming calm.

Thursday 1:30 P.M.	20 min	When I started the exercise, I felt restless and agitated. My thoughts were racing, and I kept going over work stuff. This made me more frustrated at first and I had thoughts like "I can't do this" and "I'm wasting my time." I practiced accepting these thoughts and feelings, rather than fighting them, and returned my attention to my breathing. I was able to keep practicing.
Friday 11:55 A.M.	3 min	I could only do a few minutes between clients, but it was helpful in setting me up for my next session (I noticed I was more able to be present).
Sunday 5:00 P.M.	15 min	I spent most of the exercise lost in thought (worries and planning for the coming week) but was able to be patient with myself.

Over the next week, try to practice 5 out of 7 days. In terms of the duration of your practice, start small and build up to between 10 and 20 minutes. As in Erica's example above, practicing for only a few minutes can have a powerful effect on your day. You might want to experiment with the timing of your practice: for example, before or after a therapy session, first thing in the morning, or as you return home from work.

There are common obstacles that can arise when beginning a mindfulness practice. Such obstacles can be both internal and external: from new-brain thoughts about "getting it right" or feeling bored or restless, to the time limitations created by child care or a busy working life. You can, however, use such obstacles as opportunities to relate mindfully to your experiences: Notice the kinds of thoughts and feelings you encounter as you consider or undertake your practice. People commonly become frustrated when they notice their thoughts taking them away over and over again—but becoming distracted in this way is an important part of mindfulness training, because it helps us learn to notice movement in the mind. Bringing mindful awareness to such obstacles allows us greater clarity about how best to work with such experiences or situations (for example, to consider ways to help ourselves remember to do the practice), and to compassionately consider our various needs and responsibilities. This process also provides us with a demonstration of compassionate coping: Instead of avoiding our struggles, we look deeply into them with the intention of understanding the causes and conditions that create and maintain them, asking, "What would be helpful as I work with this obstacle?"

In the third column, note any experiences you observed in doing the exercise. These might include thoughts and feelings about doing the practice, experiences you noticed during the exercise, and how you worked with mind-wandering, distractions, or any difficulties you encountered.

✍ EXERCISE. My Mindful Breathing Record

Day and time of practice	Duration	What I noticed

Self-Reflective Questions

What was your experience as you engaged in the mindful breathing practice? Were there any surprises? What did you learn?

_____

_____

_____

_____

_____

_____

_____

_____

_____

_____

_____

_____

_____

How did you find carrying out the mindful breathing on a regular basis? How easily were you able to complete the task daily? What obstacles arose, and how did you work with them (or how might you do so in the future)?

_____

_____

_____

_____

_____

_____

_____

_____

_____

_____

_____

_____

_____

From your experience, what might be the best way to introduce mindfulness to your clients? What might be the best way to help them develop a mindfulness practice over the course of treatment?

_____

_____

_____

_____

_____

_____

_____

_____

_____

_____

_____

_____

_____

From your experience, how do you think mindfulness relates to the CFT model? How do you think mindfulness might support and complement the cultivation of compassion?

MODULE 7

Shaped by Our Experiences

C FT differs from other approaches to self-compassion work in its emphasis on helping clients make compassionate realizations about *how things came to be this way* in their lives. In this way, clients' (and therapists') understanding of things they don't like about themselves can shift from *"something that is fundamentally wrong with me"* to *"things are uncomfortable, but are not my fault."* The "not my fault" message in CFT is really this: Let's not attack and shame ourselves for things we didn't choose or design. You've experienced some of this approach already, when Modules 2, 4, and 5 prompted you to explore one set of powerful influences on human functioning and development: our evolved brains and the tricky ways they can shape our experience. This module explores another set of influences that can powerfully shape human beings in ways we largely don't get to choose or design: the powerful manner in which we are shaped by our learning histories. Module 8 expands on this topic by helping you explore your relationship styles and how they might relate to early attachment experiences.

Shaped by Experience

For decades, behavioral psychologists have explored the ways in which social environments can shape our behavior through various learning processes such as classical conditioning, operant conditioning, and social learning (Skinner, 1953; Bandura, 1977; for an excellent contemporary discussion of behavioral principles, see Ramnerö & Törneke, 2008). Our own learning histories shape us through the positive and aversive consequences that follow the things we do and through our observation of the behviors modeled by others. Over time, our environments are teaching us what behavior is acceptable and will lead to desirable outcomes, and what behavior is unacceptable and will be followed with punishment. Although such consequences are usually anchored to our observable behavior, they can also shape how we relate to our private experiences, such as thoughts and emotions, through the rewarding and punishment of our verbal and nonverbal expression of these experiences (e.g., emotional responses or talking about what we think). We also learn from our observations of others' behavior—which behaviors they model for us (from which we learn what sorts of behavior are acceptable) and which behaviors they do not (for example, the emotions they never express—which can teach us that certain emotional experiences are unacceptable). In this way, we learn to experience some behaviors, thoughts, and emotions as things that are good about us, and we learn to relate to other behaviors, thoughts, and emotions with rejection, self-criticism, and shame. The tricky nature of our evolved brains will lead most of us to experience a wide array of thoughts and emotions that we are not necessarily choosing to have, which can create problems for us. To add to these difficulties, our threat-focused old brains are very good at linking together experiences and emotions which can condition us to have powerful, unchosen reactions to various experiences (for example, having powerful emotional reactions to various sensory cues that were present during a traumatic experience in the past). We are powerfully socially shaped.

In this section, you'll explore a bit about how your own learning history has shaped you. In preparation, let's take a look at Joe's example.

 EXAMPLE: Joe's Reflection

> **Growing up—at home, school, and in your other environments—what did you learn about how you should behave? What ways of behaving did you learn were desirable (e.g., behavior you were rewarded for or which you saw modeled by others), and what ways were deemed undesirable (e.g., behavior for which you were punished or ridiculed, or which were never modeled by your caregivers)?**
>
> *Growing up, I learned that I was supposed to be productive and do things according to the rules. I learned that there is a right way to do things, and that is how they're supposed to be done. I also learned that it's important to be honest and to do your best to help others when they need it—I guess that's why I became a therapist. In terms of what you're not supposed to do, I learned that one is supposed to be polite and agreeable—it's not OK to brag or to be rude. My father was quick to criticize me, sometimes harshly, if I didn't comply or if he thought I was being lazy, and my teachers were sort of like that as well.*
>
> **Growing up—at home, school, and in your other environments—what did you learn about what and how you should feel (for example, by observing emotions that were expressed by your caregivers)? Did you learn anything about what types of feelings were acceptable and unacceptable?**
>
> *It sounds so stereotypical to say this, but as a male I really did learn that somehow it was OK for me to feel and express anger, but not "weaker" emotions like anxiety or*

sadness. My father would often model anger to me—raising his voice and the like, never physically aggressive—but he never really showed anxiety or sadness, and was quick to shut it down in me if he saw me looking scared or tearful. And, of course, the other boys would come at you mercilessly if they saw any of that. So I learned to shut that stuff down pretty quickly. I guess I don't really express many of my emotions, honestly, but anger is easier, although it makes me uncomfortable because it reminds me of the parts of my father that I don't want to emulate.

Growing up—at home, school, and in your other environments—what did you learn about what and how you should think? Did you learn anything about what types of thoughts were acceptable and unacceptable?

I think maybe that I learned to not trust my own judgment a little bit—you know, to just go along and do what I'm told even if it doesn't seem quite right to me. That has created some challenges for me when I've been in situations like the one I'm in at work right now—where the things people were telling me about how I should do something didn't fit with what I think is right, or with my values. I've also learned that it's bad to be arrogant, or to have cruel thoughts—so sometimes I find myself appalled by the things that enter my head. As a therapist, I know that people will have all sorts of thoughts, so that's not really a problem for me. The real issue is finding a way to assert myself when my judgment conflicts with those above me.

As you were growing up, did you learn anything about compassion and how to relate to suffering in yourself and others?

Well, there was a general message that you should help others who need it, although we never really talked about compassion. My parents did donate to the local food bank, and I think there was a volunteer project at school a time or two. But most of the time, our family mostly just did our stuff . . . focusing on the daily tasks of life. With regard to my own suffering, it sort of relates to what I wrote above—there wasn't really any focus on what to do with that from my father, except for a general dismissing of feelings like fear or sadness. My mother was a little different; when she could see I was upset, she'd come to me, give me a hug, and tell me it would be all right. It's nice to remember that. So as I think about it, I guess she did teach me that when people are hurting, it is important to show them you care about them. Maybe that's why I ended up becoming a therapist.

In the following exercise, reflect on how you've been shaped by your environment through rewards and punishments, and through life experience. It might be good to find a comfortable place where you won't be disturbed for a bit, and to take a few moments to engage in some soothing rhythm breathing to engage your parasympathetic nervous system and prepare for self-reflection.

EXERCISE. Exploring What I've Learned

Growing up—at home, school, and in your other environments—what did you learn about how you should behave? What ways of behaving did you learn were desirable (e.g., behavior you were rewarded for or which you saw modeled by others), and which were deemed undesirable (e.g., behavior for which you were punished or ridiculed or which were never modeled by your caregivers)?

Growing up—at home, school, and in your other environments—what did you learn about what and how you should feel (for example, by observing emotions that were expressed by your caregivers)? Did you learn anything about what types of feelings were acceptable and unacceptable?

Growing up—at home, school, and in your other environments—what did you learn about what and how you should think? Did you learn anything about what types of thoughts were acceptable and unacceptable?

As you were growing up, did you learn anything about compassion and how to relate to suffering in yourself and others?

Self-Reflective Questions

How was it reflecting on the learning experiences that have shaped your current behavior, emotions, and thinking? What feelings arose?

_____

_____

_____

_____

_____

_____

_____

_____

_____

_____

_____

_____

_____

Did you notice any obstacles or resistance? If so, how did you understand and work with them?

_____

_____

_____

_____

_____

_____

_____

_____

_____

_____

_____

_____

_____

_____

Did you notice any compassion arising—or reluctance to experience compassion—as you considered how your life experiences have shaped your current ways of being in the world?

_____

_____

_____

_____

_____

_____

_____

_____

_____

_____

_____

_____

_____

From your experience of these exercises, what considerations do you feel should be borne in mind when introducing these ideas to clients?

_____

_____

_____

_____

_____

_____

_____

_____

_____

_____

_____

_____

_____

Compassionate Functional Analysis

In this module, we consider the ways in which humans can be shaped by our experience in relation to a problematic situation. This exercise involves bringing to mind an example of the challenging problem you identified in Module 1. We guide you through a typical behavioral functional analysis—identifying the antecedents, observing the behavior (which can include even private events such as thinking or emotional responses), and noting the consequences that follow—which will help you identify the triggers, typical patterns, and conditions that tend to maintain the problem. Then we prompt you to compassionately consider how your response in this situation makes sense within the context of your history and the current conditions that surround it. This part of the process involves considering how your experience of this problem might have been shaped by your past, and how your experience and responses make sense within that context, as Joe does next.

 EXAMPLE: Joe's Reflection

Briefly describe a recent example of the problem.

My situation was a typical one at my new job. During a staff meeting, we were trying to staff our new intakes and do some treatment planning around them, and our unit supervisor seemed oblivious—he kept hammering us on our productivity requirements and emphasizing how important it is that we keep our schedules full even to the point of suggesting double-booking. He seemed uninterested in talking about the clients and how to help them.

Is there something in your response to the situation that you find problematic? This can be an outward behavior, an internal behavior such as a thought, or even an emotion with which you feel uncomfortable. It might be something that you are ashamed of or for which you criticize yourself.

Well, I think I was right to be frustrated. It just seems like the focus isn't where it should be. But I guess I am a bit ashamed that not only didn't I say anything at the meeting, instead I stewed about it all day, which distracted me from thinking about my clients. I even was a bit snappish at my family when I got home, which is not OK to me.

What aspects of the situation triggered your response? It could be something that happened, an aspect of the context you were in, or even another of your feelings and emotions—anything that provoked this particular response in you.

No guessing there—it was my supervisor's attitude. He just doesn't seem to get it.

Now, consider the consequences of your response. What happened afterward? How might these consequences have rewarded or punished your response in ways that made it more likely to either happen (or to not happen) in the immediate future and/or in the long term?

I guess I could divide the consequences of my response into the short term and longer term. In the short term, not saying anything probably helped me avoid getting into a confrontation with my supervisor in the meeting, which wouldn't be fun at all. However, stewing about it all day kept me from enjoying my day, probably kept me from doing my best work with my clients, and got in the way of my being present for my family in the way I want to be. And being able to observe that led to some self-criticism, as I became aware that I was acting in a way that wasn't very helpful over all.

Reflecting on your response in relation to your own learning history as well as in relation to the current situations that trigger it and the consequences that follow it, does it make sense that you would struggle with this situation? Knowing what you know about yourself and how you learned to be in the world, does it make sense that you might behave, feel, or think in this way when faced with this situation? How might your reaction have been shaped by factors you didn't choose or design?

As I think about it, it really does make sense. Growing up, I was expected to follow my father's requests without question—and if I did question him, his response could be really harsh. So I could see how I learned to keep it inside for fear of creating a big conflict. At the same time, I saw him model the very thing I was doing this week—stewing over what he was upset about and snapping at us rather than addressing the problem. And that helps explain why I'm so hard on myself about it, because it's hard to watch myself acting in ways that were so hard for me to watch when I was growing up—there are a lot of things about my father that I admire, but not that stuff.

EXERCISE. My Functional Analysis

Now explore your own challenging situation, considering relationships between your responses to the situation and previous learning experiences that may have shaped your tendencies to respond in particular ways.

Briefly describe a recent example of the problem.

Is there something in your response to the situation that you find problematic? This can be an outward behavior, an internal behavior such as a thought, or even an emotion with which you feel uncomfortable. It might be something that you are ashamed of or for which you criticize yourself.

What aspects of the situation preceded or triggered your response? It could be something that happened, an aspect of the context you were in, or even another of your feelings and emotions—anything that provoked this particular response in you.

Now, consider the consequences of your response. What happened afterward? How might these consequences have rewarded or punished your response in ways that made it more likely to either happen (or to not happen) in the immediate future and/or in the long term?

Reflecting on your response in relation to your own learning history as well as in relation to the current situations that trigger it and the consequences that follow it, does it make sense that you would struggle with this situation? Knowing what you know about yourself and how you learned to be in the world, how does it make sense that you might behave, feel, or think in this way when faced with this situation? How might your reaction have been shaped by factors you didn't choose or design?

Self-Reflective Questions

Did the functional analysis make sense to you? Did anything in it not feel right? What did you learn about yourself through this exercise (e.g., about how you were shaped by your previous experience and the factors maintaining your experience in the here and now)?

_____

_____

_____

_____

_____

_____

_____

_____

_____

_____

_____

Did you notice any fears, obstacles, or resistance? If so, how did you understand and work with them?

_____

_____

_____

_____

_____

_____

_____

_____

_____

_____

_____

_____

Did you notice any compassion coming up in you (or reluctance to experience compassion) as you considered how your life experiences have acted to shape how you engage with this problem?

_____

_____

_____

_____

_____

_____

_____

_____

_____

_____

_____

Does anything stand out that might inform how you approach this process with your clients? Can you think of any clients for whom this exploration might be helpful? How might you use it with them?

_____

_____

_____

_____

_____

_____

_____

_____

_____

_____

_____

_____

How does your experience of the last two modules relate to your understanding of the CFT model? How might such exercises be used to facilitate compassion in clients?

_____

_____

_____

_____

_____

_____

_____

_____

_____

_____

_____

_____

_____

Safe-Place Imagery

Previously, we introduced the three affect regulation systems (threat, drive, and soothing/safeness) and discussed how the new brain and old brain can interact to activate these systems and create momentum around particular affective and motivational states. We also learned about how breathing in certain ways can help bring the physiology of the soothing system online. In this module, we continue to explore ways of working with inputs to the emotional brain to get the soothing system online, to balance our emotions, and to help ourselves shift into compassionate motivational states—setting the stage for us to engage actively and compassionately with challenging experiences and emotions.

A Brief Introduction to Imagery

In this module, we introduce our first imagery practice. Sometimes people struggle with imagery, believing that it must involve the creation of vivid images in the mind, which some people can find very challenging. The way we use imagery in CFT isn't as much about creating picture-perfect mental photographs as it is about creating *mental experiences* that facilitate felt shifts in understanding, emotion, and motivation (Gilbert, 2010; Kolts, 2016). To demonstrate this process, let's do a brief experiential exercise:

1. First, bring to mind waking up and getting up this morning. What did you notice first? How did you feel in your body? What sounds did you notice? Notice your first movements out of bed: Where were you heading? What did you notice on the way—and when you get there? What sounds, sights, smells, and tastes presented themselves to you as you oriented to the day? Do you recall any felt sense in your body as you got going in the morning?

2. Second, bring to mind a favorite food. Explore this experience in your mind. What does this food look like? Taste like? What's its texture? What else do you notice about it? Its smell? The memories it conjures? Notice the mental experience that takes shape as you bring this food to mind—both the sensory information coming in (sights, sounds, etc.) as well as the level of motivation, interest, or enjoyment that you experienced while eating this food.

3. Third, bring to mind a recent vacation or holiday you've taken (or, perhaps one you'd like to take). Try to get a mental sense of this place—the atmosphere, the temperature, the feel of the air on your body. The sights? The sounds? The smells? The colors? What's it like? What would it be like to be there? How would it feel? What do you notice? How do you feel recalling this?

Let's take a moment to reflect on what we learned in going through this exercise. Whether or not you were able to create vivid images of each suggested experience, were you able to create a *mental* experience that corresponded to the prompt? What did you notice?

 EXAMPLE: Joe's Imagery Practice

What I noticed during the imagery practice:
I experienced myself opening my eyes to the sound of the alarm, beeping loudly. My body felt warm and heavy and I felt these sensations as I imagined them, with the weight of the covers on me. It surprised me that I felt a bit tired and sleepy doing the exercise, and I wanted to go back to bed!

What I learned during the imagery practice:
I learned that imagery can create the same kind of feelings as if I were back in that moment. Even though I couldn't really see it like a vivid picture, I got a clear sense of it—I could imagine the alarm and I really felt its sound in my body. It also made me want to do certain things, like return to bed.

 EXERCISE. My Imagery Practice

What I noticed during the imagery practice:

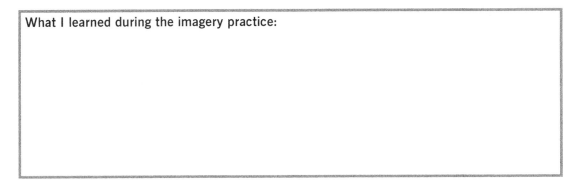

What I learned during the imagery practice:

Getting the Safeness System Online through Imagery

In CFT, a primary goal of therapy is to help our clients get their safeness/soothing systems online and working for them. To help our clients do this, it's important to learn how to facilitate feelings of safeness in ourselves as well. The safeness system gives us a powerful way to help balance out feelings of threat so that we can be at our best in working with challenging emotions and life situations. However, depending upon our inherited temperaments and how we've been shaped by life experiences (see Modules 7 and 8), some of us can have underdeveloped safeness systems and may struggle to bring up feelings of safeness in ourselves. Other people may experience very specific blocks that inhibit their ability to access experiences of soothing and calm, or may even experience reluctance around trying to bring up these experiences in themselves. Over time, we want to help ourselves and our clients develop a repertoire of behaviors and strategies that will give us the ability to activate, develop, and strengthen our safeness systems, so that we grow increasingly able to stimulate these feelings in ourselves over time—even in the face of more and more challenging experiences. Let's begin by introducing an imagery practice designed to do just this: safe-place imagery (Gilbert, 2009).

EXERCISE. Safe-Place Imagery

As we did in the preceding exercise, we're going to use imagery to create experiences in the mind—but this time, we use imagery to create a soothing input to the old, emotional brain to help get that safeness system working for us.

Let's start by doing a minute or so of soothing rhythm breathing, slowing down the breath, using the body to slow down the mind. Recall that in doing this, we aim for a rhythm of around six breaths per minute, inhaling for 4–5 seconds, perhaps holding for a moment, and then slowly exhaling over a space of 4–5 seconds. If it would be helpful, take a moment to revisit the soothing rhythm breathing practice described in Module 3.

Once we've slowed things down in our bodies and minds, let's begin to imagine what it might feel like to feel completely safe, completely content, and completely at peace. What might these pleasant experiences feel like in our bodies?

In this practice, we use imagery to construct a mental "place" that will bring these feelings up in us. Let's do that now. You might read through the following instructions and then close your eyes and do the exercise.

- Bring to mind the sort of place that might bring up feelings of safeness, peace, and content-edness in you. This might be a place you've visited in the past, or it might be a completely imagined place that you develop based on things that you know help you feel safe.
- As you bring this place to mind, consider the sensory details of this place. Take some time for each one:
  - What do you see?
  - What do you hear?
  - What do you smell?
  - What is your bodily experience (e.g., the warm feeling of sun on your skin)?
- Notice the emotions that come up as you focus on these various details. If there are particular aspects of this place that bring up powerful feelings of peacefulness, contentedness, or safe-ness, perhaps focus on those and build from there.
- There may or may not be other people or beings (e.g., animals, supernatural beings) in this place with you. If there are, imagine that these beings are welcoming—delighting in your pres-ence, glad that you are here. Play around here with distance—maybe the other person, people, or beings are nearby. Or maybe they are somewhere in the periphery of the image. Focus on whatever is helpful for you.
- Imagine that this place itself welcomes you—that it is pleased you are here and appreciates your presence, as if you complete it.
- It's very common in the beginning to find ourselves shifting from place to place until we settle on one. It's also common for people to imagine several different "places" they might visit, depending upon what feels right at the moment. The point is the *process*—the goal of learning how to bring up feelings of safeness—and connecting with a particular mental place or image that helps to elicit those feelings. Feel free to experiment to find "places" that work for you.
- Spend some time enjoying this place. You may wish to start by spending 5 minutes or so in the beginning (feel free to take longer). When you are ready, take a few soothing breaths, open your eyes, and return to the day, bringing some of that sense of peace and safeness back with you. Write a bit about your experience of the practice, as Fatima has below:

 EXAMPLE: Fatima's Safe-Place Imagery

Day of practice	Experience of safe-place imagery practice	Reflections on the practice
Day 1	I was anxious as I shut my eyes and started the practice—my mind was racing and I thought I wouldn't be able to manage more than a minute. But the breathing helped and I was able to picture a quiet beach, feel the warm sand on my feet, and hear the waves. I felt calm and content.	I was quite resistant to doing the exercise and had put off starting. It's that threat of slowing down, wondering what will I find. I could feel my body changing, but this took time. . . .

EXERCISE. My Safe-Place Imagery

Day of practice	Experience of safe-place imagery practice	Reflections on the practice

Self-Reflective Questions

Was there anything that surprised you about your experience of safe-place imagery?

_____

_____

_____

_____

_____

_____

_____

_____

_____

_____

_____

_____

_____

_____

Did you experience any blocks to the exercises? If so, how did you understand and work with them?

_____

_____

_____

_____

_____

_____

_____

_____

_____

_____

_____

_____

_____

Did you arrive at any new insights about the soothing/safeness system during the exercise? If so, what were they?

_____

_____

_____

_____

_____

_____

_____

_____

_____

_____

_____

_____

_____

_____

Are there any implications that you can draw from your experience and take into your therapy practice?

_____

_____

_____

_____

_____

_____

_____

_____

_____

_____

_____

_____

_____

_____

From your experience, are there any implications for your understanding of how safe-place imagery impacts on the threat, drive, and safeness systems?

_____

_____

_____

_____

_____

_____

_____

_____

_____

_____

_____

_____

MODULE 10

Exploring Attachment Style

In Modules 7 and 8 you reflected upon how your learning history has shaped your current experience—your tendencies to experience certain emotions, thoughts, and behaviors—as well as how you respond to these tendencies (e.g., with pride or shame). In this module, we explore another aspect of our learning histories that can powerfully shape our lives—our attachment histories and current attachment styles.

Shaped by Our Relationships

Module 2 introduced the three-circles model of emotion. The soothing/safeness system functions to help us access experiences of calm and peacefulness, helping us regulate our emotions and work with experiences of threat. For decades, attachment theorists have characterized the attachment behavioral system—the ways in which we are able to connect with and be soothed by contact with others—as being core in helping us respond to threats in a healthy fashion and having the confidence to explore the world and our own emotions (Bowlby, 1969/1982; Wallin, 2007; Mikulincer & Shaver, 2007). Our early attachment experiences powerfully shape how we experience others (as helpful, caring, and present—or not) and ourselves (as worthy of love and caring—or not), as well as providing us with a model of how to respond to ourselves and others when we are in distress.

Attachment insecurity (involving ongoing tendencies to relate to interpersonal relationships with anxiety, avoidance, or both) has been the focus of thousands of scientific studies. It has been linked with a wide range of life difficulties, including depression, anxiety disorders such as posttraumatic stress disorder (PTSD) and obsessive–compulsive disorder (OCD), personality disorders, and eating disorders (Mikulincer & Shaver, 2007, 2012), as well as with difficulties experiencing self-compassion (Pepping, Davis, O'Donovan, & Pal, 2014; Gilbert, McEwan, Catarino, Baião, & Palmeira, 2014). Relevant to CFT, the facilitation of attachment security—the ability to readily engage with and feel safe in relationships with others—has been linked with a range of positive outcomes, such as increases in self-confidence and self-development (Feeney & Thrush, 2010); self-compassion (Pepping et al., 2014); as well as compassion, empathy, and altruistic behavior (Mikulincer et al., 2001; Mikulincer & Shaver, 2005; Gillath, Shaver, & Mikulincer, 2005). The point is increasingly made that therapists can act as a secure base to help clients regulate in the face of threat and in assisting them to approach and work with difficult experiences (Wallin, 2007; Knox, 2010; Kolts, 2016).

Given all of this research supporting the importance of attachment relationships, it may not come as a surprise that attachment histories, styles, and dynamics in the therapy room are important in CFT. In the rest of this module, you'll explore your own attachment experiences and how they have shaped the ways in which you relate to other people and to yourself. Looking deeply into our own attachment histories and how they've shaped our current lives can sometimes bring up a surprising level of emotion, as these dynamics are often at the heart of the experiences that we find to be most difficult. So as you complete the exercises in this module, make sure to *take care of yourself*—if possible, give yourself time to do the exercises in a quiet, comfortable space, and perhaps plan a pleasant activity to do afterward.

Let's start by revisiting the brief attachment questionnaire from Module 1, which will help you get a sense of how much you tend to experience attachment anxiety and avoidance. As we've noted before, the direction of the numbers changes in the middle of the measure—we've done this because the first four items are reverse-scored. All you need to do is circle the response that best fits your experience and then sum your scores.

ECR-RS

Please read each of the following statements and rate the extent to which you believe each statement best describes your feelings about **close relationships in general**.	Strongly disagree						Strongly agree
1. It helps to turn to people in times of need.	7	6	5	4	3	2	1
2. I usually discuss my problems and concerns with others.	7	6	5	4	3	2	1
3. I usually talk things over with people.	7	6	5	4	3	2	1
4. I find it easy to depend on others.	7	6	5	4	3	2	1
5. I don't feel comfortable opening up to others.	1	2	3	4	5	6	7
6. I prefer not to show others how I feel deep down.	1	2	3	4	5	6	7
7. I often worry that others do not really care about me.	1	2	3	4	5	6	7
8. I'm afraid that other people may abandon me.	1	2	3	4	5	6	7
9. I worry that others won't care about me as much as I care about them.	1	2	3	4	5	6	7

Attachment Avoidance (sum items 1–6): _____
Attachment Anxiety (sum items 7–9): _____

Attachment avoidance scores range from 6 to 42, with higher scores indicating a greater tendency to avoid or feel uncomfortable around relating closely with others. Attachment anxiety scores range from 3 to 21, with higher scores indicating tendencies to experience anxiety around relationships and the extent to which others care about you or the possibility that they might abandon you. Now let's consider a few other questions that will help you explore your attachment experiences and how these experiences have shaped you. In this exercise, we focus on a few questions:

- Growing up, to whom did you feel close?
- What did you do when you were upset? Were your parents or caregivers able to help you feel safe and calm down?
- In your present life, what are your relationships like? Do you have close relationships with others in which you feel accepted and safe? Is it easy or difficult for you to feel close to others?
- In your present life, what do you do when you are upset? Are you able to turn to others for support? Is connection with others helpful to you when you're experiencing distress?

Fatima and Erica decided to complete this exercise as a limited co-therapy pair, using Socratic questioning to explore Fatima's attachment tendencies, while embodying compassionate qualities such as kind curiosity, empathy, and steadfast support. Chapter 4 contains a description of working in limited co-therapy pairs. In the following excerpt, Erica has taken the role of the therapist.

 EXAMPLE: Exploring Attachment

ERICA: In this module, we're exploring attachment tendencies—looking at our early relationships and how they've shaped us. How are you feeling about doing that?

FATIMA: A bit apprehensive. My relationship with my parents wasn't the smoothest, so it isn't the easiest thing to think about, but I think it will be helpful. Let's go ahead and dive in.

ERICA: (*Smiles.*) I really appreciate your courage. We'll go ahead, but let's make sure to pay attention to how you're feeling as we proceed. To whom did you feel close when you were growing up?

FATIMA: To be honest, there weren't that many people. I had a couple of fairly close friends, and in my family, my grandmother was probably the person I felt closest to. In high school, I had a group of girlfriends that I really enjoyed spending time with as well. That was really nice, because in junior high I had felt set apart sometimes because I was the only Pakistani kid in the class—it felt like they just didn't really know what to make of me. That didn't seem to be as much of an issue in high school.

ERICA: I'm sorry to hear about your not fitting in because of your ethnicity—I imagine that was really tough for an adolescent girl.

FATIMA: At times it really was. At that age, you just want to fit in, you know? I've always been proud of my Pakistani heritage, and I love so many aspects of my culture, but sometimes I've wished I was just like everyone else—just because it would have made things easier. . . . (*Pauses.*) And then I'd feel ashamed of that, like I was betraying my family and my culture by thinking it.

ERICA: (*Pauses.*) Thanks so much for sharing that, Fatima—it felt really honest and vulnerable. It sounds like you felt caught between wanting to fit in and valuing your heritage. Looking back, does it make sense that this adolescent version of you might have struggled with those feelings?

FATIMA: (*Pauses thoughtfully.*) It does, you know? All adolescents want to fit in, so of course I would have struggled with that. (*Pauses and then smiles gently.*) It feels good to say that. Thanks!

ERICA: (*Smiles.*) You're welcome. Ready for the next question?

FATIMA: Sure.

ERICA: Could you tell me what you did when you were upset? Was your family able to help you calm down and feel safe in those times?

FATIMA: (*Pauses.*) This feels kind of uncomfortable, because I don't want to speak ill of them, but my parents weren't always so helpful when I was struggling. My mother struggled with depression, so she wasn't always reliable. My father tried, but he seemed kind of clueless—it just seemed hard for him to understand the things that girls go through. I appreciated his making the effort, though. Both of them could get pretty critical and controlling, so if I turned to them, I wasn't sure what would happen—whether I'd get supported or be blamed and criticized for being upset. For example, when I mentioned the racist experiences I'd had at school, they told me it was important to just ignore it when that happened and not make a fuss if someone made comments about my color—that this was what they'd had to do when they first arrived in this country. So when I needed support, I'd be more likely to turn to friends. My grandmother was the most helpful—she'd make some tea, get out some sweets, let me talk it out, and tell me that everything was going to be alright. (*slightly teary*) Those were really nice times.

ERICA: (*Smiles tenderly.*) What a beautiful image I have of you and your grandmother, there together. It must have been hard for you to feel unable to turn to your parents. I'm glad your grandmother could be there for you in that way.

FATIMA: Yeah, I didn't get to see her as often as I would have liked, but the time we did spend together was really special.

ERICA: (*Pauses.*) It sounds like it. Could you talk about what your relationships are like in your current life? Do you have relationships in which you feel safe and accepted? Is it easy for you to feel close to others?

FATIMA: I have a few friends that I feel close to—friends from my university. When I scored the questionnaire, I fell right in the middle on both the anxiety and avoidance scales—not too low or high. I think these scores relate to one another, in that I tend to be anxious that others won't be interested in me or care about me, which leads me to keep some distance—both in terms of doing things with others and in sharing what I'm feeling. It's not terrible, though. Some of my clients struggle with this so much worse than I do—at least I have some close friends.

ERICA: So you've noticed that you tend to keep some distance from others, maybe because you've learned that those who are close to you won't always be helpful when you're having a hard time?

FATIMA: Yes, I think that's it.

ERICA: Given what you've told me about how your parents responded to your distress growing up, does it make sense that you might respond in that way?

FATIMA: It completely makes sense. I'm really appreciating the way you're listening to me right now—you're really good at this! (*Smiles.*)

ERICA: (*Smiles.*) Thanks. I've really enjoyed getting to know you better through conversations like this, which really underscores the point that these sorts of connections are helpful. I think I heard you say that although you sometimes tend to distance yourself from others, you're able to connect with friends—you said you have some close ones?

FATIMA: Yes, that's right—although it might be helpful if I reached out to them more often.

ERICA: We've sort of moved on to the next set of questions: In your present life, what do you do when you are upset? Are you able to turn to others for support? Is connection with others helpful to you when you're experiencing distress?

FATIMA: (*Pauses.*) Hmm . . . I think it varies for me right now. I talk with my parents sometimes, but that's just catching up; I don't bring up difficult topics. They're not so supportive of my career, and they keep telling me about how well the kids of their friends are doing at their jobs and asking me when I'm getting married. So they're not helpful when I'm struggling, and it can feel like they're more concerned with how my struggle reflects upon them rather than the fact that I'm having a hard time. I sometimes call my college friends to chat. My friend Susan is a psychologist as well, so she can really sympathize about the work-related problems that come up. But it's tough sometimes because I don't want to be a burden—I don't mind chatting about life generally, but it's hard to share when I'm having a problem. Sometimes I feel really isolated, like I don't have anyone to talk to about it. (*Pauses.*)

ERICA: So it can be hard for you to reach out, even when it might be helpful to you, because you don't want to be a burden?

FATIMA: Yeah, it's always felt more comfortable for me to be the helper than the one who's being helped. It's probably part of the reason I became a therapist.

ERICA: That makes a lot of sense to me.

FATIMA: I've started journaling sometimes after seeing how helpful it was for a couple of my clients, and that's seemed to help when I remember to do it.

ERICA: That's a great idea. So that's been helpful?

FATIMA: It has. At least it helps me get out of my head and get my thoughts straight.

ERICA: And you said earlier that you thought it might also be useful to reach out to friends more often. Is that something you think might help when you find yourself struggling?

FATIMA: I think so. When I've reached out in the past, they've been really helpful. I think the problem has been my willingness to do that.

ERICA: In the workbook, it talks about three flows of compassion—compassion for others, compassion for ourselves, and our ability to receive compassion from others. It sounds like you may have some reluctance around that third flow—giving yourself permission to receive caring from others. Does that fit for you?

FATIMA: It really does. That was a higher score for me on the questionnaire we did in the first module as well.

ERICA: So it sounds like receiving compassion from others might be an area of growth for you to work on?

FATIMA: It won't be easy, but I've been thinking the same thing the past few minutes. Thanks. This has been really helpful. (*Smiles.*)

ERICA: (*warmly*) Thank you, Fatima.

Now, taking a few minutes to consider your own attachment history and the way it plays out in your current relationships, reflect on the following questions, either alone or in conversation with a partner:

 EXERCISE. Exploring My Attachment History

In this exercise, you'll reflect on your attachment experiences, both growing up and in your present life.

Growing up, to whom did you feel closest?

Growing up, what did you do when you were upset? Were your parents, caregivers, or other people able to help you feel safe and to calm down?

In your present life, what are your relationships like? Do you have close relationships in which you feel accepted and safe? Is it easy or difficult for you to feel close to others?

In your present life, what do you do when you are upset? Are you able to turn to others for support? Is connection with others helpful to you when you're experiencing distress?

In CFT, there's the recognition that we evolved to feel safe through connection with others who accept us and care about us (Gilbert, 2010). As we've seen, however, our ability to do this can be complicated by developmental factors that may have taught us that others may not be available—or reliably helpful—when we're in distress. In this way, the therapy room can be like a laboratory in which some of our clients learn to experience relational safeness with another person for perhaps the first time.

Self-Reflective Questions

Exploring one's attachment history can be quite challenging. Was it challenging for you? If so, how? Did anything catch you unaware and surprise you?

_____

_____

_____

_____

_____

_____

_____

_____

_____

_____

_____

How do you think that your own attachment history and current style might influence you as a therapist with clients or as a supervisee in supervision?

_____

_____

_____

_____

_____

_____

_____

_____

_____

_____

_____

_____

Reflecting on your experience of these exercises, does anything stand out that might inform how you introduce ideas about attachment history to your clients? From what you have experienced, what kinds of considerations might arise about when, with whom, and how to introduce attachment ideas?

_____

_____

_____

_____

_____

_____

_____

_____

_____

_____

_____

From your experience of this module, what sense do you make of the relationship between attachment theory and the CFT model?

_____

_____

_____

_____

_____

_____

_____

_____

_____

_____

_____

_____

MODULE 11

Exploring Fears of Compassion

In Module 10, you explored your attachment history and considered how your early relationships with caregivers might impact your current relationships, and in particular, what you do when you find yourself struggling. This discussion is particularly relevant to the development of compassion, because that's exactly what compassion is about: what we do when we encounter suffering and struggle in ourselves and other people, including our clients. CFT focuses on how this compassion can manifest in three "flows": compassion that is directed outwardly to others, compassion that is offered to ourselves, and compassion that is directed to us from others.

Depending upon our histories, we may find ourselves feeling really good about connecting with some of these compassionate flows, while having great difficulty with others. For example, we've met a number of other therapists who excel at experiencing and enacting compassion for vulnerable others, even as they struggle to treat themselves kindly when they're struggling, or in allowing others to take care of them when they need it. Paul Gilbert called these difficulties "fears of compassion" (FOC; Gilbert, 2010; Gilbert, McEwan, Catarino, Baiao, & Palmeira, 2013) and with his colleagues, operationalized them in the form of the FOCS (Gilbert et al., 2011).

If we're going to help our clients access these flows of compassion, it's necessary to explore our own ability to do so. You've got a head start on that, having answered a few of the questions from the FOCS in Module 1, along with a few items we've adapted for this book. To frame the work in this module, let's revisit those questions, filling out the items below and summing them, as indicated, to find your subscale scores for the three flows. It's important to keep in mind that the items below are just a sampling of a few items from the FOC scale, combined with a few summary items developed for this book (the full, validated scale was too long to include in this book). It hasn't been validated, so please don't use it with clients or in research—you can download the full, validated scale at *https://compassionatemind.co.uk/resources/scales*.

FOCS ITEMS

Please use this scale to rate the extent to which you agree with each statement.	Do not agree at all		Somewhat agree		Completely agree
1. Being too compassionate makes people soft and easy to take advantage of.	0	1	2	3	4
2. I fear that being too compassionate makes people an easy target.	0	1	2	3	4
3. I fear that if I am compassionate, some people will become dependent upon me.	0	1	2	3	4
4. I find myself holding back from feeling and expressing compassion toward others.	0	1	2	3	4
5. I try to keep my distance from others even if I know they are kind.	0	1	2	3	4
6. Feelings of kindness from others are somehow frightening.	0	1	2	3	4
7. When people are kind and compassionate toward me, I "put up a barrier."	0	1	2	3	4
8. I have a hard time accepting kindness and caring from others.	0	1	2	3	4
9. I worry that if I start to develop compassion for myself, I will become dependent upon it.	0	1	2	3	4
10. I fear that if I become too compassionate toward myself, I will lose my self-criticism and my flaws will show.	0	1	2	3	4
11. I fear that if I am more self-compassionate, I will become a weak person or my standards will drop.	0	1	2	3	4
12. I struggle with relating kindly and compassionately toward myself.	0	1	2	3	4

Note. This adaptation involves a limited selection of items from the FOC scale as well as additional summary items developed for this book. It was developed so that readers of this book could have a brief way of tracking their progress in working through the modules. As such, this selection of items has not been validated and is not appropriate for use in either research or clinical work. Readers can acquire a copy of the complete, validated version of the scale which is appropriate for research and clinical purposes at *https://compassionatemind.co.uk/resources/scales.*

Adapted from Gilbert, McEwan, Matos, and Rivis (2011). Copyright © 2011 The British Psychological Society. Reprinted with permission from John Wiley & Sons, Inc., in *Experiencing Compassion-Focused Therapy from the Inside Out: A Self-Practice/Self-Reflection Workbook for Therapists* by Russell L. Kolts, Tobyn Bell, James Bennett-Levy, and Chris Irons. Published 2018 by The Guilford Press. Permission to photocopy this form is granted to purchasers of this book for personal use only (see copyright page for details).

> Fears of Extending Compassion (sum items 1–4): _____
>
> Fears of Receiving Compassion (sum items 5–8): _____
>
> Fears of Self-Compassion (sum items 9–12): _____

Filling in the items from the FOCS might have given you a sense of which flows of compassion are more and less comfortable for you. Let's explore this area in a little more depth by reflecting upon the scores from the scales. Take a few minutes for yourself in a quiet space; perhaps engage your soothing rhythm breathing, and reflect upon the ways in which you are able to connect with compassion, and the ways in which you may struggle to do so.

 EXAMPLE: Fatima's Reflection

> **Reflecting on your scores on the FOCS items, what did you notice? Which flows of compassion are more and less comfortable for you? How do you make sense of that?**
>
> I noticed that although my problems have centered on this particular client with whom I've struggled—and for whom I've struggled to have compassion—that my challenges really seem to be focused on having compassion for myself and receiving it from others. On the subscale for receiving from others, although my scores overall weren't that high, I noticed that I seem to keep myself distant from others somewhat out of fear that they will find out something about me that will drive them away, and perhaps from reluctance to face my own emotions. In terms of compassion for myself, it seems that I use criticism to motivate myself, and that I have some resistance to stopping that and feeling self-compassion instead—like I'm reluctant to give up the criticism for fear of losing my edge. I think I'm also scared of problems that could arise if I do have compassion for myself—my score on the "becoming dependent upon it" question was pretty high. Maybe I'm worried to find myself relying upon something that I won't be able to sustain, or of having to face feelings that make me uncomfortable.
>
> **What feelings and thoughts do you have as you reflect on your responses to the scales?**
>
> A bit of surprise, but also some relief. I've been worried lately about this reaction I've had to this client—I've always experienced myself as having compassion for others, but I have really struggled with her. That's bothered me a lot. These scales seem to reflect me as I liked to think of myself before—being very willing to be compassionate toward others, even as I sometimes struggle to receive it for myself. I guess I'm more comfortable with that somehow, even though I know I need to develop these other flows. I'm also aware that I'm not as motivated to develop compassion for myself, as if having compassion for myself isn't as important as having it for others. Both of these may relate to a general reluctance to face my own uncomfortable feelings and explore them—something I've never really been good at. That's something I need to work on, although like I said, it's hard to motivate myself to do that. I need to find a way to convince myself that I matter, too, and to have the courage to face my feelings even when they're uncomfortable.

Take a moment to reflect upon your own responses to the scale. Looking at the scale sums and any particular items you may have scored highly on, consider if there are areas in which you generally struggle more with compassion than others. Consider what you've noticed about how you connect with the three flows of compassion—which ones feel natural, and which ones are more challenging for you. You may notice that these tendencies relate to the attachment experiences you explored in Module 10.

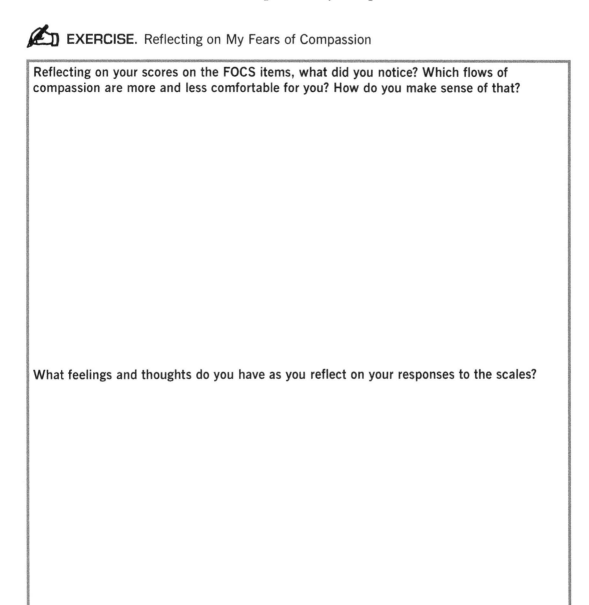 **EXERCISE.** Reflecting on My Fears of Compassion

Reflecting on your scores on the FOCS items, what did you notice? Which flows of compassion are more and less comfortable for you? How do you make sense of that?

What feelings and thoughts do you have as you reflect on your responses to the scales?

Self-Reflective Questions

Did anything surprise you or concern you in doing the FOCS items? Did you have any new insights? If so, what were they?

_____

_____

_____

_____

_____

_____

_____

_____

_____

_____

_____

_____

_____

How valuable do you think it would be for your clients and for yourself to use the FOCS in therapy? When might you choose to do so—or not?

_____

_____

_____

_____

_____

_____

_____

_____

_____

_____

_____

_____

_____

_____

Threat-Focused Formulation in CFT: Historical Influences and Key Fears

In CFT, a threat-based formulation focuses on—as the name suggests—the nature of the threats we experience. The formulation particularly focuses on how these threats developed, efforts to manage them in the here and now (i.e., safety strategies), and how these strategies can lead to a number of unintended consequences that can negatively impact our lives. Finally, the formulation explores how these unintended consequences, via sensitizing certain types of self-to-self relating styles (e.g., self-critical) and further distress, may create feedback loops by fueling current fears and threats rather than addressing them (Gilbert, 2009, 2010). In these next two modules, we explore the different aspects of the formulation. This module covers the first two elements: historical influences and key fears and threats.

Historical Influences

The formulation begins with an exploration of our historical experiences and emotional memories. As we introduced previously in Module 7, we're looking for experiences that might have sensitized or shaped the threat, drive, and soothing systems. This module will especially focus on experiences and emotional memories that link to the threat system. Some of us will have histories involving trauma or difficult attachment experiences, but there are many other sorts of experience that can shape our threat responses in tricky ways. These could be experiences with parents, siblings, or extended family. They could include experiences with friends, peers, or even a romantic partner. They might also include common experiences linked to pursuing goals, such as trying to do well academically or in the workplace.

Key Fears and Threats

The next step of the formulation involves helping clients consider how their experiences have shaped their threat systems in the here and now. Many of our fears are archetypal: As humans, there are certain common themes that cause us distress, such as rejection, abandonment, isolation, shame, and harm (Gilbert, 2010). In CFT, we also distinguish between external threats and internal threats. External threats involve the outside world (e.g., other people), such as fears of being rejected, abandoned, disliked, or criticized by others. Internal threats involve fears around how we relate to our own experience, such as fears involving our own emotions (e.g., fears of becoming overwhelmed by sadness, anxiety, anger, or by feeling vulnerable or alone), memories (e.g., of past trauma, shame memories, or mistakes), or concerns about our identity (e.g., a shame-based identity that involves experiencing oneself as weak, inferior, or flawed). Let's consider Fatima's formulation, which she and Erica decided to explore via a limited co-therapy dyad:

 EXAMPLE: Exploring Fatima's Historical Influences and Key Fears

ERICA: Fatima, you had volunteered to go first with the threat-based formulation. Is that still all right?

FATIMA: Certainly. Having looked through the module, I know we'll be getting into some personal stuff, but we've done that before, and I feel safe with you. Let's do it.

ERICA: That's wonderful to hear. We'll go ahead and get started then. The formulation begins with looking at historical influences—things in our past that have shaped the way our threat systems respond. It looks like this includes memories that have uncomfortable emotions or shame attached to them. Want to start with your family environment?

FATIMA: Sure. (*Pauses to think.*) You know some of this already. (*Pauses.*) Things at home were challenging growing up. I really looked up to my father, and sometimes he was really warm and sensitive, you know, but he was unpredictable.

ERICA: (*Nods.*) Could you talk a bit about that?

FATIMA: Everything could seem fine, and then he'd just become super controlling and critical. It seemed like whatever I did, however well I did in school, it wasn't good enough. (*Pauses thoughtfully.*) A lot of the time, he was just gone. I'm not sure if it's because he was so wrapped up in his work, or because things were so bad with Mom, but I remember him being gone more than he was there. It made me feel like he didn't care about me. Mom seemed depressed, and she could get really distant and irritable. She and Dad fought a lot, and I think she initiated much of that because she was so unhappy. Looking back, it seems like she was caught between cultures—between this image in her mind of the good Pakistani wife that she thought she should be, and the models of the American women she saw on TV and around her—which she seemed to envy and hate at the same time. It's like she'd hold it all in until she started drinking, and then blow up. They separated when I was 12. After that, I lived with Mom, but was mostly on my own.

ERICA: (*Pauses.*) That sounds really hard.

FATIMA: It was. The time I spent with my grandmother helped—but I didn't get to see her very often.

ERICA: You mentioned that you got the sense that however well you did in school, it wasn't good enough. Could you talk a bit about what things were like at school?

FATIMA: Sure. I worked hard in school—my parents really emphasized that it was important to succeed academically, and how expensive it was to send me to private school. I remember at age 13, I had this moment of thinking that if I could only do well enough and get straight A's at school, maybe my parents would be so happy at how good and successful I'd become that they'd get back together again. That didn't happen, and I felt like nothing I could do would make them love me and each other, so I sort of gave up. Socially, I had some good friends, which was really nice—but as I mentioned before, I also had some experiences of racism.

ERICA: Would you mind telling me a bit more about that?

FATIMA: Well, I was the only kid of Pakistani descent in my school, so sometimes the kids would make fun of me and call me racist names. And after 9/11, people seemed a lot more paranoid of people who look different or "un-American." Once I was approached by a group of girls and one of them called me a terrorist and then slapped me. I fell down crying. It was humiliating.

ERICA: Fatima, that sounds terrible. I'm so sad that happened to you.

FATIMA: It was pretty awful. It still bothers me when I think about it. At the time, I was sort of in shock about it, and I didn't know what to do. It made me feel ashamed to be who I am. (*Pauses, thinking.*) It's better now. The past few years I've really embraced my culture and I'm proud of my Pakistani heritage. But back then I just wished I could be like everyone else. I did have a lovely group of friends during much of my schooling, but it was hard to feel safe and trust that they really liked me. I remember when I'd hear that my friends had done something without me—gone to a game or something—I'd feel really alone and rejected, even though they were just doing their thing.

ERICA: Has that part gotten better?

FATIMA: It has, but as I've told you, I've tended to keep my distance in some ways. I've been working on connecting with friends more as we've gone through this process, and it seems to be helping. But it's an effort—my default is to avoid getting too close.

ERICA: That sounds like a safety strategy. We'll get to that later, but it seems like a good way to transition to key fears. What fears do you think you were trying to protect yourself from with that distancing?

FATIMA: I've always been afraid of rejection—like underneath everything, there was this sense that I wasn't good enough, and that if people really got to know me, they'd see that and wouldn't want to have anything to do with me. Related to that, I've had fears that people would turn on me, finding something they didn't like about me and then criticize me and attack me for it.

ERICA: (*Pauses.*) Fatima, that sounds really hard for you, feeling like if you really shared who you are, that you'd be criticized and rejected.

FATIMA: (*Pauses.*) It was. (*Looks down at her hands.*)

ERICA: (*Pauses, looking kindly at Fatima.*) Given what you've told me about how critical your parents could be, and some of the experiences you've had of being bullied, does it make sense that you would have these fears?

FATIMA: It does. (*Pauses.*) It really does. I spent a lot of time lost in books, trying to feel anything other than what I was feeling. I went to see a therapist at 15, which helped. She helped me realize that a lot of this wasn't my fault, and she was really patient with me even when I tried to push her away. She's why I ended up becoming a therapist myself.

ERICA: I'm glad you had her.

FATIMA: I am, too.

We continue with Fatima's formulation in Module 13. For now, you can see how the preceding information was summarized on Fatima's CFT Case Formulation Worksheet (on page 122).

FATIMA'S CFT CASE FORMULATION WORKSHEET

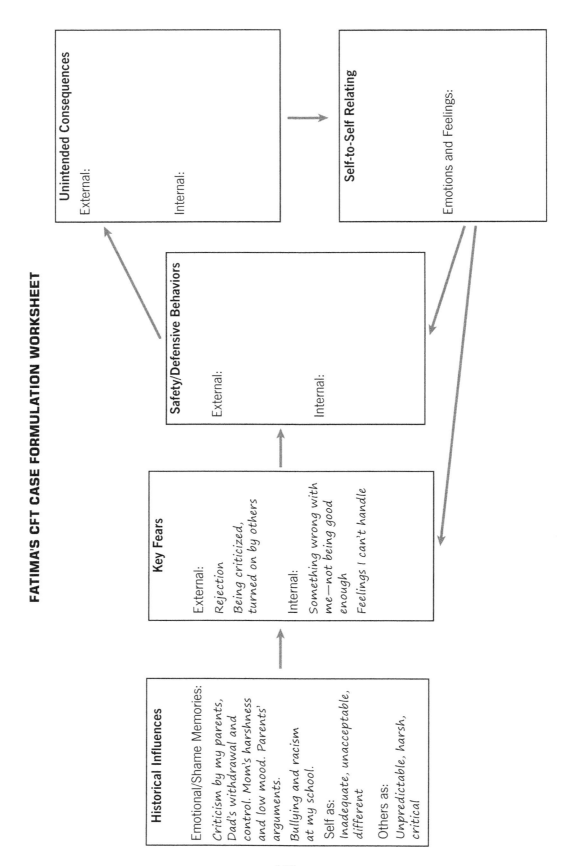

Historical Influences

Emotional/Shame Memories:

*Criticism by my parents,
Dad's withdrawal and
control. Mom's harshness
and low mood. Parents'
arguments.
Bullying and racism
at my school.*

Self as:

*Inadequate, unacceptable,
different*

Others as:

*Unpredictable, harsh,
critical*

Key Fears

External:

*Rejection
Being criticized,
turned on by others*

Internal:

*Something wrong with
me—not being good
enough
Feelings I can't handle*

Safety/Defensive Behaviors

External:

Internal:

Unintended Consequences

External:

Internal:

Self-to-Self Relating

Emotions and Feelings:

Take some time to consider these first two columns in your own formulation. As with the previous exercises, try to find some time in which you can be undisturbed for a few minutes. Find a quiet space to reflect upon the experiences in your life and how they may have shaped fears in you relating to the world and other people, and in how you relate to your own emotions and self-identity. When you're ready, answer the reflective questions in the following exercise or in your own journal.

 EXERCISE. Exploring My Historical Influences and Key Fears

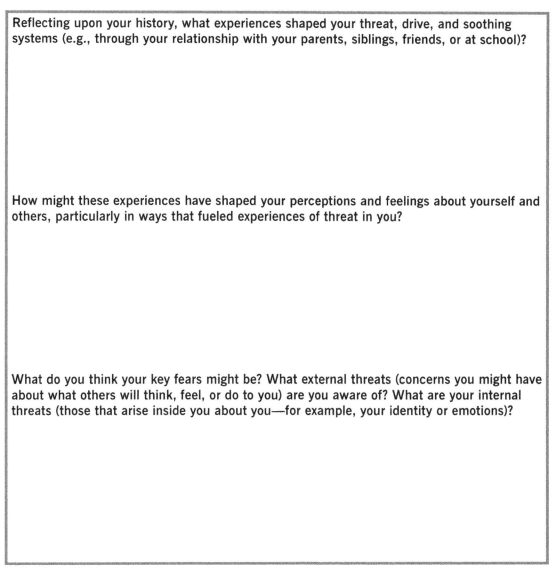

Reflecting upon your history, what experiences shaped your threat, drive, and soothing systems (e.g., through your relationship with your parents, siblings, friends, or at school)?

How might these experiences have shaped your perceptions and feelings about yourself and others, particularly in ways that fueled experiences of threat in you?

What do you think your key fears might be? What external threats (concerns you might have about what others will think, feel, or do to you) are you aware of? What are your internal threats (those that arise inside you about you—for example, your identity or emotions)?

As Fatima did, you can also summarize your information in the CFT Case Formulation Worksheet (on page 124).

MY CFT CASE FORMULATION WORKSHEET

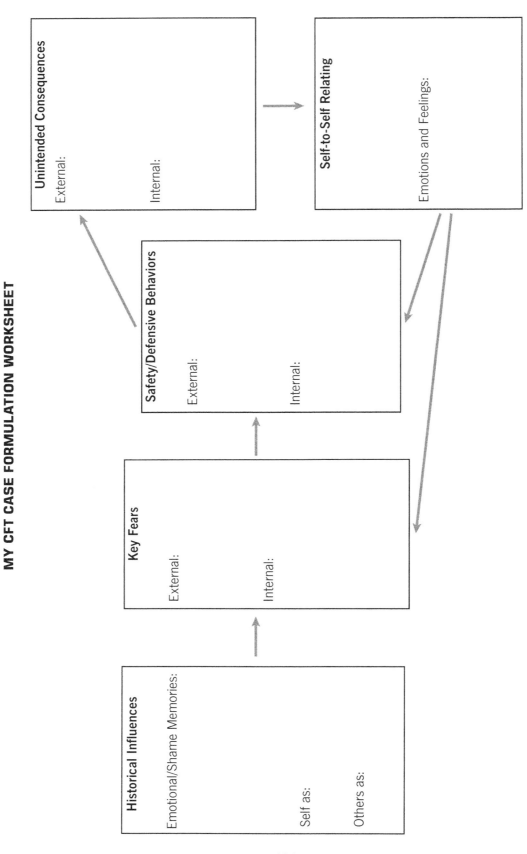

Historical Influences

Emotional/Shame Memories:

Self as:

Others as:

Key Fears

External:

Internal:

Safety/Defensive Behaviors

External:

Internal:

Unintended Consequences

External:

Internal:

Self-to-Self Relating

Emotions and Feelings:

Technique Tip: Sometimes our clients (or even we) can struggle to identify key fears. One efficient strategy for doing so comes from CBT, in the form of David Burns's (1980) *downward-arrow* technique. With the downward arrow, we start by identifying something that is bothering the individual in his or her daily life—perhaps represented by what CBT therapists might call an "automatic thought." Starting with this thought or fear, we then ask, "Why is this so upsetting to you? What does it mean?" To get at internal fears specifically, the second question can be asked as "What does it mean *about you*?" When the answer comes, the same questions are asked again. Repeating this process through a few iterations will typically lead us straight to the key fear, often signaled by a surge in emotion (or in clients, nonverbal behavior signaling an emotional response). Once you've gotten to the key fear, Socratic questions can be used to link the fear to your own or the client's history, as in Joe's following example.

 EXAMPLE: Joe's Downward Arrow

I snapped at my wife and daughter again last night.
Why is this upsetting? What does it mean?   *I shouldn't do that. They don't deserve to be treated like that.*
Why is this upsetting? What does it mean?   *It means I was doing a terrible job as a husband and father.*
Why is this upsetting? What does it mean?   *Maybe I __am__ a terrible husband and father.*
Does this fear—that you're a terrible husband and father—does that fear make sense when we think about it in terms of your history? Can you see how you might have acquired this fear?   *Yeah. My father was often critical of me and pointed out when I would screw things up— and this is what's most important to me, so of course I'd be afraid of messing it up.*

 Self-Reflective Questions

What was your experience of considering your history and key fears? What emotions or bodily experiences did this exercise bring up in you?

_____

_____

_____

_____

_____

_____

_____

_____

_____

_____

_____

_____

_____

If you experienced reluctance to continue or subtle avoidance at any stage of the process, how did you work with it?

_____

_____

_____

_____

_____

_____

_____

_____

_____

_____

_____

_____

Did you feel any compassion (or not) when considering your historical experiences, key fears, and how these might be related?

_____

_____

_____

_____

_____

_____

_____

_____

_____

_____

_____

_____

_____

_____

Reflecting on your own experience of these exercises, what are the implications for your work with your clients? How might you introduce the formulation diagram?

_____

_____

_____

_____

_____

_____

_____

_____

_____

_____

_____

_____

_____

_____

_____

Does your experience of this aspect of the formulation make sense in terms of your understanding of the CFT model? Are you left with any questions?

_____

_____

_____

_____

_____

_____

_____

_____

_____

_____

_____

_____

_____

_____

Threat-Focused Formulation in CFT: Safety Strategies and Unintended Consequences

In Module 12, you explored the first two elements of the threat-based formulation: formative historical influences, and key fears and threats. Many clients present to therapy with problems related to these core threats and how they've attempted to work with them. Often, these efforts will have involved using strategies that have produced unhelpful unintended consequences (Gilbert, 2010). In CFT, these efforts are often called "safety strategies," and tend to involve efforts to reduce acute contact with uncomfortable threat experiences. Hence, such strategies often tend to involve either active or passive avoidance. Examples include the socially anxious individual (perhaps harboring a good deal of shame about aspects of him- or herself that he or she is afraid others will see, and fearing rejection) who avoids relationships, or the individual who struggles with anger, but blames others for his or her outburst. Both of these strategies serve to limit immediate contact with a threat (the social situation or the realization that the person has a problem with anger), but ultimately produce unintended consequences that can be crippling, and which, over time, can negatively shape the individual's experience of him- or herself and others (Gilbert, 2010). As we did in Module 12, let's briefly explore these aspects of the formulation.

Safety, Protective, and Compensatory Strategies

Like other animals, when threatened, humans engage in a variety of strategies in the attempt to manage and cope. These strategies are often linked to evolved behavioral responses—for example, seeking protection from others, moving away from (flight/

avoiding) others, aggression (fight), or submission (freeze)—and can be anchored to either external or internal threats (Gilbert, 2009, 2010). These strategies often develop in childhood or adolescence, and can become elaborated and reinforced via conditioning processes into adult life.

Unintended Consequences and Self-to-Self Relating

Because of their often-reactive and avoidant nature—focused on limiting contact with perceived threats in the short term with no consideration of the long term—safety strategies typically have unintended maladaptive consequences. It's important to help clients—and ourselves—recognize that these consequences are *unintended*—we don't set out to engage in behavior that will ultimately make our lives worse. Moreover, in the short term these strategies are often experienced and described as at least somewhat helpful in managing threats. However, such consequences can often impact the ways we relate to ourselves (e.g., as weak, incompetent, unlikeable, bad, or flawed in some way) and to others (e.g., as untrustworthy, judgmental, or to be avoided) (Gilbert, 2010). In turn, these consequences can then lead to the development or maintenance of unhelpful self-to-self styles of relating, which can produce distress, trigger further safety strategies, and reactivate or fuel our key fears. A feedback loop is likely to develop, in which the system reinforces itself over time, preventing natural correction.

Let's reconnect with Fatima and Erica as they explore these portions of Fatima's formulation.

ERICA: Fatima, you've told me a bit about your key fears, which seem focused on the anticipation of being criticized and rejected, of not being good enough, and perhaps of being afraid of your own emotions. (*Points to CFT Case Formulation Worksheet.*) Does that sound right to you?

FATIMA: (*Pauses, looks down.*) Yes, that sounds right.

ERICA: (*Leans in a bit.*) Could you tell me how you're feeling right now?

FATIMA: It's just . . . it's just that it feels both hard and kind of a relief to see it down on paper. It's hard to admit that the experiences I had growing up left me with these fears, but it feels validating to finally say it: "I'm really afraid of rejection." "I'm really afraid that there's something wrong with me." It's also hard to admit to myself how much of my life has been driven by those fears.

ERICA: (*Pauses.*) It sounds like you're really putting some things together right now. You mentioned that parts of your life have been driven by your fears—that sounds like safety strategies, which is the next part of the formulation. Could you talk a little more about that?

FATIMA: For starters, I think the fears have impacted how I relate to other people. My parents could be so critical that I just stopped sharing things with them, which sort of generalized to other people. Even with friends, I've always been much more of a listener than a talker, and I find ways to not share information about myself.

ERICA: Would you say that you try to avoid criticism by not sharing yourself with others—by not providing them with information about you that they could criticize?

FATIMA: Exactly. It's like "What they don't know can't hurt me." (*Chuckles a bit.*)

ERICA: (*Smiles.*) That makes sense to me, and I can see how that could help you avoid the situations you fear. Has this strategy led to any unintended consequences?

FATIMA: Yes, I think it has—I've found it often stifles my relationships. I've had people tell me that I'm "hard to get to know." I guess there was always a part of me that felt like I wasn't worth knowing. I think that's why I also tend to avoid social opportunities. Don't get me wrong—I do have friends, and some fairly close ones. But I tend to avoid social opportunities that involve being around new people and going too deeply in the relationships I already have.

ERICA: How has that pattern impacted your life?

FATIMA: It's hard to know, but at a practical level it's meant that I haven't done much professional networking. I get notification of these meetings for newer therapists and young professionals, and never end up going. I know that networking is helpful in terms of getting referrals and other opportunities, but I just haven't done much of it. I also haven't done much dating, which is something I'd like to do, but it is really intimidating.

ERICA: So you tend to avoid anything that involves really opening up to others?

FATIMA: Yes—that makes me feel really vulnerable, so I tend not to do it. I can be quite a homebody.

ERICA: I'm wondering if there are any other strategies you've used to try and cope with those fears.

FATIMA: (*Pauses thoughtfully.*) In school, I worked really, really hard to get good grades, and that's translated into my job as well. It feels very important that I be able to help my clients. A lot of that is that I do have compassion for them and their struggles, and I want to help them, but I think part of that is about me as well.

ERICA: Like you're trying to prove something to yourself?

FATIMA: Maybe. Or maybe disprove something. It's like, behind everything is this fear that I shouldn't be doing this—that I don't have what it takes. Even when I look at the things I do well, that fear is still there.

ERICA: Given the experiences you had growing up, does it make sense that this fear would linger?

FATIMA: It does. But it's tough, because every time I struggle with a client, it triggers my threat system and that self-critical part of me shows back up again. So I end up perseverating about whether or not I have what it takes to be a good therapist rather than on how I can best help my clients—which I'm pretty sure makes me a less effective therapist.

ERICA: That sounds tricky.

FATIMA: It is. Of course, I know deep down that all therapists will struggle sometimes, and that clients will have ups and downs during therapy. But even knowing that, I'm learning that the downs trigger my fears, and then I end up ruminating.

ERICA: Would you say that ruminating about those fears is another safety strategy? Like if you keep thinking about whether or not you're a good therapist, it will somehow make you a better one?

FATIMA: (*Smiles.*) It sounds ridiculous, but I think that's exactly what I do.

ERICA: If it's all right, I'd like to summarize now, because you've given me a lot of information about your safety strategies and their unintended consequences.

FATIMA: Sounds good.

ERICA: It sounds like you've coped with your fears of criticism and rejection by not really opening up to others—first with your parents and then more generally—and that maybe the unintended consequence of that safety strategy has been having fewer and perhaps less meaningful relationships. Does that sound right?

FATIMA: (*Nods.*) It does.

ERICA: I think I also heard you say that you avoid social opportunities that might be helpful—networking opportunities and even dating—with the result that you miss out on potential opportunities and relationships that might contribute to your life.

FATIMA: Mmm-hmm.

ERICA: Finally, you didn't use the term *perfectionism*, but it seems like there is a flavor of that—like maybe you cope with this fear of not being good enough by working really hard to do a good job at school and work, and then by ruminating over it and criticizing yourself when you struggle and don't meet your high expectations.

FATIMA: (*Nods.*) That's right.

ERICA: On the worksheet under fears, we also have "feelings I can't handle." Do you think you have any safety strategies around those?

FATIMA: I think it's more of what we've been talking about. As we've gone through the modules, I've realized that up until now, I haven't really paid much attention to my feelings. I don't usually share them with others, and even when I'm on my own, I busy myself with work, reading, housework, and activities like taking my dog for a walk. But I don't pay much attention to my feelings, maybe because I'm afraid of getting lost in them. Like if I go there, I won't be able to get back.

ERICA: Do you think there are any consequences to avoiding your emotions in that way?

FATIMA: (*Smiles.*) Nothing ever gets resolved! The avoidance keeps me trapped where I am. It seems so stupid, now that I look at it on paper. I'm doing all this avoidance that keeps me from working through these scary feelings that I haven't even acknowledged having. As a therapist, I can look at all this and say, "I'm avoiding." I need to *do* something about that.

ERICA: It seems like, for a moment there, the self-critical version of you showed up, calling you stupid . . . but then it seemed like your compassionate self took over, orienting toward what might be helpful to address this issue. I've been reading ahead a bit, if you can't tell. (*Smiles.*)

FATIMA: (*Laughs a bit.*) Yeah. It won't be easy, but I'm feeling a bit more optimistic.

ERICA: That's great, Fatima. The last part of the formulation has to do with how all of this—particularly the safety strategies and their consequences—has shaped your relationship with yourself. Could you talk about that?

FATIMA: Well, as I look at it now, it seems pretty clear that pulling back socially and not sharing about myself have only strengthened my sense of myself as not being good enough and have fueled my self-criticism. I talk about this with my clients all the time—when we avoid social relationships, it prevents us from having good interactions that can help us feel differently.

ERICA: And get that safeness system going.

FATIMA: Yeah. Also, I think the perfectionism fits in there too. Setting standards that I can never meet pretty much makes it impossible for me to feel better about how I'm performing.

ERICA: (*Smiles and nods.*) You've really got the hang of this formulation business. What about the emotional avoidance you were talking about? How does that shape how you relate to yourself?

FATIMA: (*Pauses.*) For me, avoiding the emotions keeps me from being comfortable with them—but they're part of me, you know? (*Pauses, thoughtfully.*) So I think that kind of avoidance may feed into the idea that I'm not good enough or that there's something wrong with me—because I can't even handle my own feelings.

ERICA: (*Smiles gently.*) Feelings can be pretty hard to handle sometimes.

FATIMA: They sure can. But I can do better. I really can.

Let's take a look at Fatima's completed formulation worksheet (on page 134).

FATIMA'S COMPLETED CFT CASE FORMULATION WORKSHEET

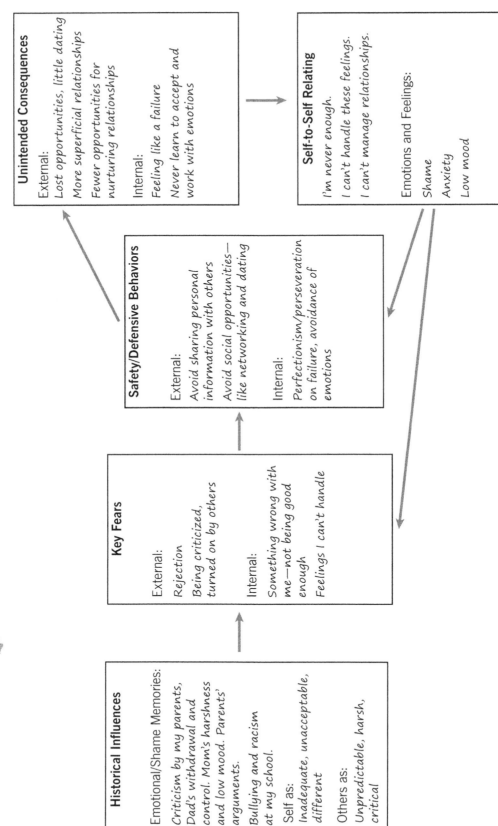

Historical Influences

Emotional/Shame Memories:

Criticism by my parents, Dad's withdrawal and control. Mom's harshness and low mood. Parents' arguments.
Bullying and racism at my school.

Self as:
Inadequate, unacceptable, different

Others as:
Unpredictable, harsh, critical

Key Fears

External:
Rejection
Being criticized, turned on by others

Internal:
Something wrong with me—not being good enough
Feelings I can't handle

Safety/Defensive Behaviors

External:
Avoid sharing personal information with others
Avoid social opportunities—like networking and dating

Internal:
Perfectionism/perseveration on failure, avoidance of emotions

Unintended Consequences

External:
Lost opportunities, little dating
More superficial relationships
Fewer opportunities for nurturing relationships

Internal:
Feeling like a failure
Never learn to accept and work with emotions

Self-to-Self Relating

I'm never enough.
I can't handle these feelings.
I can't manage relationships.

Emotions and Feelings:
Shame
Anxiety
Low mood

Hopefully the conversations between Fatima and Erica have given you a sense of how such an exploration might play out in a limited co-therapy dyad, as well as how you might facilitate such a conversation with a client. If you are doing the program on your own, you'll once again want to find a quite space where you can be undisturbed for a little while, spend a few moments doing some soothing rhythm breathing, and then review what you've written about your history and key fears in Module 12. When your responses are fresh in your mind, consider the following reflections.

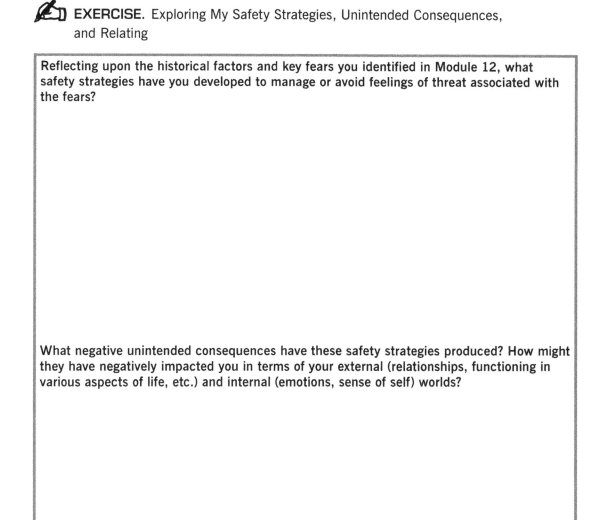

EXERCISE. Exploring My Safety Strategies, Unintended Consequences, and Relating

Reflecting upon the historical factors and key fears you identified in Module 12, what safety strategies have you developed to manage or avoid feelings of threat associated with the fears?

What negative unintended consequences have these safety strategies produced? How might they have negatively impacted you in terms of your external (relationships, functioning in various aspects of life, etc.) and internal (emotions, sense of self) worlds?

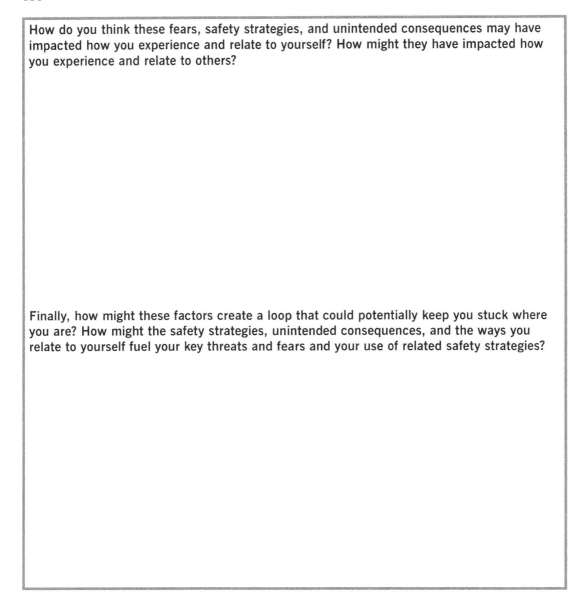

How do you think these fears, safety strategies, and unintended consequences may have impacted how you experience and relate to yourself? How might they have impacted how you experience and relate to others?

Finally, how might these factors create a loop that could potentially keep you stuck where you are? How might the safety strategies, unintended consequences, and the ways you relate to yourself fuel your key threats and fears and your use of related safety strategies?

Now that you've completed all aspects of the four-column formulation, you might find it helpful to concisely summarize your formulation on the CFT Case Formulation Worksheet (on page 137).

MY CFT CASE FORMULATION WORKSHEET

Historical Influences

Emotional/Shame Memories:

Self as:

Others as:

Key Fears

External:

Internal:

Safety/Defensive Behaviors

External:

Internal:

Unintended Consequences

External:

Internal:

Self-to-Self Relating

Emotions and Feelings:

137

Self-Reflective Questions

Were you able to identify your safety strategies easily, or was this difficult? Did they make sense? What about the unintended consequences and their link with the ways you relate to yourself and others? How useful was this way of formulating these factors in relation to your understanding of yourself?

_____

_____

_____

_____

_____

_____

_____

_____

_____

_____

_____

_____

_____

Were there any obstacles that came up as you did the formulation? If so, how did you work with them?

_____

_____

_____

_____

_____

_____

_____

_____

_____

_____

_____

_____

_____

_____

_____

As you did the formulation, did you experience any compassion for yourself? What do you make of that?

_____

_____

_____

_____

_____

_____

_____

_____

_____

_____

_____

_____

_____

_____

_____

_____

How do you think you might use this kind of formulation with clients? Can you anticipate any problems? How might you address them?

_____

_____

_____

_____

_____

_____

_____

_____

_____

_____

_____

_____

_____

_____

The Mindful Check-In

Building the habit of mindful awareness is important in CFT, and it's a capacity that can take a while to develop. In Module 6, you were introduced to mindful breathing. This module will acquaint you with the mindful check-in, a brief practice that allows us to quickly connect with our bodily experience, emotions, and thoughts.

What Is a Mindful Check-In?

The mindful check-in involves bringing attention to your experiences in a sequential manner (as described in the exercise on page 142). The check-in is a time to bring non-judgmental, mindful awareness to your experiences as they occur in a real-life setting (Kolts, 2011). This practice aims to bridge the gap between formal meditation (such as mindful breathing) and a mindful awareness of our daily lives as we interact with other people and go about our clinical work. In this way, the practice aims to cultivate the *habit* of mindfulness. It is also a helpful dipping-in point for individuals who could benefit from mindful awareness but who may be resistant to the idea of engaging in meditation.

Learning to Notice the Mind and Body

As we've discussed in earlier chapters, our emotions and motivations powerfully organize the mind: grabbing our attention, coloring our thinking, and guiding our behavior. The aim of the mindful check-in practice is to help us get to know these processes in real time, so that we can learn to notice the first stirrings of our emotions, as well as our habitual reactions to particular stimuli. Ultimately, the practice is designed to help us reduce our "mindless" acting out of emotions, motivations, and old patterns of thought and behavior, while providing us with an opportunity to choose how we would like to respond to our immediate situation and experiences. In the mindful check-in, you'll start by bringing your attention to your bodily experience, gradually moving it to your thinking, your emotions, your motivation, and then to your reactions to the exercise itself.

 EXERCISE. Mindful Check-In Practice

1. **What I notice in my body:**
   - *What do I feel in my body?*
   - *Am I tensed or relaxed? How can I tell? Where do I feel it?*
   - *What sensations are prominent?*
   - *What is the temperature of my body?*
   - *What are the contact points of my body with the outside world (e.g., feet on the floor)?*
   - *What is my body posture? How am I sitting or standing?*

2. **What I notice in my emotions:**
   - *What emotions do I feel?*
   - *What emotional tone am I experiencing? Can I give my feelings an emotional label?*
   - *Is there more than one emotion? Which emotions stand out?*

3. **What I notice in my thinking:**
   - *What am I thinking? What are the contents of my thoughts (what are they about?)?*
   - *What images or pictures come to mind?*
   - *What is my thought process like? Are my thoughts fast or slow, narrowly focused or reflective?*

4. **What I notice I want to do (impulse to act):**
   - *Is there anything I want to do right now?*

5. **What I notice in my reactions:**
   - *What are my reactions to the exercise?*
   - *When noticing the thoughts, feelings, emotions, or impulses I experience, do I have any strong reactions?*
   - *Do I have any additional thoughts about what I've found going on in my mind or body?*
   - *Am I making any judgments or criticisms?*
   - *Do I notice judgments—thinking that certain experiences are right or wrong?*
   - *Are any experiences wanted or unwanted?*
   - *Do I notice wanting to do anything about what I've found in my experiences?*
   - *What thoughts arise in relation to particular emotions or body sensations, or vice versa?*

Let's take a look at Erica's Mindful Check-In Record:

EXAMPLE: Erica's Mindful Check-In Record

Day of the week/time	What I noticed when I mindfully checked in with myself (body sensations, thinking, emotions, impulses to act, and reactions)
Monday 1:00 P.M.	I notice I'm tense across my shoulders and neck and I'm thinking, "I'm too tired to see any more clients." I feel stressed and fatigued. I'm aware there's a real pull to go home and go back to bed. I also notice judgments about what I'm feeling: "I shouldn't be feeling this" and "There must be something wrong," which make me feel a bit anxious.

Because a primary challenge for our clients (and ourselves) when it comes to a practice like this one is remembering to do it, it helps to come up with a plan. Schedule a time each day when you can realistically check in with yourself. You might consider setting an alarm on your phone or watch, or problem-solve other ways that might help you remember. After trying a few days at a set time, you could experiment with alternate times of the day. Use the following form to keep track of what you observe during your check-ins for the next week.

 EXERCISE. My Mindful Check-In Record

Day of the week/time	What I noticed when I mindfully checked in with myself (body sensations, thinking, emotions, impulses to act, and reactions)
Monday	
Tuesday	

Wednesday	
Thursday	
Friday	
Saturday	
Sunday	

✍ EXERCISE. My Mindful Check-In During Threat Activation

Once you're familiar with the mindful check-in, try using it when your threat system has been activated. This involves mindfully turning *toward* your inner experience as threat-focused emotions such as anxiety and anger are organizing your thinking, sensations, and behavioral urges. Bringing mindful awareness to your threat system in action allows you to cultivate a greater awareness of how these threat reactions play out in your life, at times when mindfulness is perhaps most difficult but also most beneficial.

The next time you notice your threat system coming "online," pause and complete the following chart. Note the situation or trigger for your experience of threat and document your experience in a non-judgmental way. As in the preceding exercise, pay attention to how you react to these experiences: for example, how anxiety-related bodily sensations might be followed by judgmental thoughts and self-criticism. See if you can bring a similar mindful orientation to any such judgments or criticism that you notice. If you struggle to remember to do the exercise during a randomly-happening threat experience, you might begin by bringing a recent threatening experience to mind and then doing a check-in in relation to the experiences that come up.

Situation/trigger for my threat reaction	What I noticed when I mindfully checked in with my threat reaction (body sensations, emotions, thinking, impulse to act, reaction)

Self-Reflective Questions

What was it like to step out of "autopilot" and check in with your experiences? Were there any surprises? What did you learn?

_____

_____

_____

_____

_____

_____

_____

_____

_____

How did you find carrying out the mindful check-in on a regular basis? How easily were you able to complete the task daily? What helped or hindered you?

_____

_____

_____

_____

_____

_____

_____

_____

_____

_____

_____

_____

What was it like to "tune in" to your threat protection reactions in a mindful way? What did you discover or learn?

_____

_____

_____

_____

_____

_____

_____

_____

_____

_____

_____

_____

From your experience, what might be the best way to introduce mindfulness to your clients? What might be the best way to help them develop a mindfulness practice over the course of treatment?

_____

_____

_____

_____

_____

_____

_____

_____

_____

_____

_____

_____

From your experience, how do you think mindfulness supports and complements the cultivation of compassion?

_____

_____

_____

_____

_____

_____

_____

_____

_____

_____

_____

Unpacking Compassion

If you look at the different measures that seek to assess compassion, you'll discover some variability from measure to measure. This is because, unlike some qualities that mental health professionals seek to measure, experiencing and acting with compassion involve a number of different psychological processes. CFT has approached this complexity by beginning with a standard definition of compassion, which itself has multiple components, and then specifically exploring the processes needed for this compassion to be experienced and skillfully applied (Gilbert, 2010; Kolts, 2016). In CFT, compassion isn't simply a value to be cultivated, it is an orientation to suffering, an answer to a question that is crucial to the world of psychotherapy: *What do we do when we encounter suffering and struggle in ourselves and others?* Throughout several of the following modules, we'll gradually unpack and explore how compassion is defined and cultivated in CFT.

Defining Compassion

In the Foreword to this book (p. vii), Gilbert presented CFT's working definition of compassion: "sensitivity to suffering in self and others with a commitment to try to relieve and prevent it." This definition highlights that compassion requires both *sensitivity*— the courageous willingness to notice and engage with suffering—as well as the *committed motivation and skills* to help do something about it. Let's do a reflective exercise to explore how you experience these aspects of compassion.

Relating to Suffering and Struggle

In the following exercise, you'll be prompted to reflect upon how you tend to engage with suffering and struggle—your own and that of other people. In doing so, you'll consider sensitivity to suffering: Do you notice suffering in yourself and others or does it tend to not show up on your "radar"? Are you moved by it, or do you tend to be numb to it? Do you tend to look deeper in order to understand it, or to ignore or turn away from it? Once you've noticed suffering, there's the further question of *What do you do about it*? How do you tend to behave in the face of suffering and struggle? Do you tend to move forward to actively work with the problem, or give up and move on to something else? Do you tend to try and soothe and encourage yourself when you notice that you're suffering (or that another person is suffering), or do you shut down or even become critical?

In the next exercise, we consider the two aspects of the CFT definition of compassion. We begin by exploring sensitivity specifically in relation to how you relate to suffering in yourself and others. First, here are Joe's reflections on how he relates to suffering.

 EXAMPLE: Joe's Reflection

Sensitivity to others' suffering: Consider how you tend to respond when others are suffering and struggling. Do you tend to notice and be aware when this happens? How do you respond?

This is a bit of a tricky question, because how would I know it if I didn't notice? But I think I get what you mean. I think the answer for me is that it depends. If I'm oriented toward noticing—paying attention for signs of suffering and struggle like I do with my clients—I think I'm good at noticing. When that happens, I feel sympathetic toward them and I want to help. But a lot of times I think that doesn't happen, because I'm not paying attention or something else gets in the way. This can show up with my family. If I come home after a long day and I'm stressed out about my job, I'm not very sensitive to their suffering, because I'm still focused on myself. It's like that threat system in the earlier modules. When that's going on for me, it can be hard to notice when others are having a hard time or need help because I'm focused on my own stuff. It's probably like that with my boss, too. He's probably stressed out about the productivity at work, but he ticks me off so much that I don't really notice or think about what he might be feeling—I just get irritated with him.

Sensitivity to your own suffering: Consider how you tend to respond when you are suffering and struggling. Do you tend to notice and be aware when this happens? How do you respond?

Ha! These questions are hard to answer. I guess I could say that I notice because I'm obviously feeling it, right? However, after doing the mindfulness modules, it's clear that there's a difference between being aware of what I'm feeling versus just being caught up in it. I think a lot of the time I just end up caught up in it, so I guess I'm not really noticing. When I do notice it, I'm not sure that the way I've tended to respond has been so helpful. Although I'm working on it, a lot of the time when I've noticed how frustrated or stressed I am, I'll either beat myself up for feeling that way or I'll fantasize about really sticking it to my supervisor—neither of which helps me feel any better.

Motivation to help with suffering: When you *do* notice and become aware of others' suffering, what do you tend to do about it? Do you find yourself approaching and helping (or wanting to approach and help), or do you do something else?

When it comes to other people, I think I'm better at this. With my clients, I work hard to understand their problems and find ways to help them. Although I've done less of this at my current job—partially due to productivity pressure—I've historically spent a good bit of time in treatment planning to make sure that what I'm doing is likely to be helpful to my clients. I think that motivation drives some of my frustration right now because I think my care has suffered as a result of these requirements.

On a personal level, I could do better at this. Again, when I come home stressed, even when I see my kids or wife struggling, I don't always do my best at helping. The other night I came home and my son was really struggling with his math homework. What I wish I'd done was to patiently sit down with him and help him learn how to do it on his own. Instead, I found myself frustrated that he was struggling—he just didn't seem to be trying very hard to understand it. I tried helping him, but eventually my wife came and took over because it was clear that I didn't have much patience with him. I feel really bad about that.

Motivation to help with suffering: When you *do* notice and become aware of your own suffering, what do you tend to do about it? Do you find yourself considering ways to help yourself with this challenge, or do you do something else?

I'm getting better at this as I go through the program, but I still find myself getting self-critical sometimes. A good example is what I wrote about above—thinking about being impatient while I was helping my son with his homework and having my wife jump in and take over. It's easy to get caught up in thoughts of being a bad father for getting frustrated with my son and having anger at my wife for intruding, and then just trying to distract myself so that I don't have to think about it. That's been a real issue for me. The social shaping module helped with this, in terms of the questions I learned to ask myself: Given what is going on at work, does it makes sense that I'd struggle with this? And of course it does. But I still want to be there for my son when he is struggling and not have conflict with my wife, so I need to do a better job at helping myself manage my work stress because that's what's driving all of that. And maybe a better job at letting her help me when I'm not at my best.

As with the other exercises, we encourage you to set the stage for this exercise by finding a nice, comfortable setting in which you can be undisturbed for a few minutes. Maybe make yourself a nice cup of tea, allow yourself to settle in, and spend a minute or two doing soothing rhythm breathing—you want to get that safeness system going so that you can reflect honestly on your experience. When you're ready, take a few moments to consider how you have tended to engage with suffering and struggle when they show up in your life and in the lives of those around you.

EXERCISE. How I Relate to Suffering and Struggle

Sensitivity to others' suffering: Consider how you tend to respond when others are suffering and struggling. Do you tend to notice and be aware when this happens? How do you respond?

Sensitivity to your own suffering: Consider how you tend to respond when you are suffering and struggling. Do you tend to notice and be aware when this happens? How do you respond?

Motivation to help with suffering: When you *do* notice and become aware of others' suffering, what do you tend to do about it? Do you find yourself approaching and helping (or wanting to approach and help), or do you do something else?

Motivation to help with suffering: When you *do* notice and become aware of your own suffering, what do you tend to do about it? Do you find yourself considering ways to help yourself with this challenge, or do you do something else?

Self-Reflective Questions

Consider your experience of this module. What did you notice as you reflected upon the ways you've tended to engage with suffering in yourself and in others? Did you have any insights that you may not have realized previously?

_____

_____

_____

_____

_____

_____

_____

_____

_____

_____

_____

_____

Did you notice any obstacles or resistance? If so, how did you understand and work with it?

_____

_____

_____

_____

_____

_____

_____

_____

What have typically been the ramifications of this way of relating to your own suffering or to that of others?

How might any insights you have gained from this module affect your work with clients?

_____

_____

_____

_____

_____

_____

_____

_____

Turning to the CFT model, how well does your experience fit with it? Anything that doesn't fit?

_____

_____

_____

_____

_____

_____

_____

_____

_____

_____

_____

_____

_____

MODULE 16

Mindfulness of Self-Criticism Diary

We're usually broadly aware of whether or not we tend to be self-critical. However, if we do tend toward self-criticism, we may often persist in a largely automatic way without even noticing that we are giving ourselves a hard time. If we *do* notice, we may try to distract ourselves in various ways, such as by blobbing in front of the television or Internet or by drinking too much. We may rarely stop to listen to that internal self-critical voice from a mindful place, in order to understand its impact on our lives. It takes *courage* to stop and listen to that voice. Courage is one of the hallmarks of compassion.

This module is about stopping and listening to the internal critic using the Mindfulness of Self-Criticism Diary (MSCD). Using the MSCD, we monitor our inner critic's activity over the course of a week and note how we feel in the face of the criticism. Then we go one step further and look at whether this critic is getting the results that it desires. In this process, we'll begin to weave in some of the compassionate attributes such as distress tolerance, nonjudgment, and care for well-being. Although this is the first appearance of the MSCD in a CFT book, it is quite consistent with the CFT approach and has proven useful in group-work.

The MSCD has superficial similarities to the thought record used in CBT (Bennett-Levy et al., 2015; Greenberger & Padesky, 2015), but its role is rather different. The purpose of both the thought record and the MSCD is to direct mindful attention toward the critical voice. However, the point of using the MSCD is not to change the critical voice or to answer it back. Rather, the purpose of the MSCD is to develop awareness around this self-critical voice, to approach rather than avoid it, and to assess whether the self-critical voice is achieving the objectives that it is apparently aiming for (e.g., Is it improving our performance? Is it helping us to feel better about ourselves? Is it increasing our well-being?).

Above all, the entries on the MSCD help to inform the functional analysis of self-criticism and the individual's problems as a whole. In turn, the functional analysis contributes to the formulation, helping to build the rationale for the development of the compassionate self, which we discuss later. The idea is to explore the criticism in context and to notice the experiences that tend to trigger it and the functions that such criticism serves in your life and in the lives of your clients.

 EXAMPLE: Erica's MSCD

Working in a co-therapy pair with Fatima, Erica completed the MSCD over the course of a week. The example on page 159 is taken from the 4th day that she had completed the diary, a Thursday. There were three diary entries on that day. By this stage, Erica was becoming attuned to noticing her self-critical voice. Although she was still frequently consumed by it, as in the first and third entries (11:00 A.M. and 9:25 P.M.), her mindfulness of the voice was increasing, and she was getting more curious about its extraordinarily negative impact on her life. On occasion, she was even starting to gain a bit of distance from it. Although it was not part of the instruction to try to change her self-critical voice, Erica recognized before she saw one of her more challenging clients, Jeff (2:50 P.M. entry), that her self-critical voice wasn't helping at all, and that if the session was to be of any help to Jeff, she needed to find some compassionate motivation for herself. She did, and she realized that it changed her—and Jeff's—experience of the session.

ERICA'S MINDFULNESS OF SELF-CRITICISM DIARY

Date/time/situation (perceived threat)	Self-critical phrase(s) I used. What was the tone of voice? Were there any images (e.g., finger pointing) or a felt sense (e.g., harshness) that accompanied the voice?	Emotions and body sensations (0–100%)	Consequences—helpful or unhelpful? How did I feel? How well did it work?
Thursday 11:00 A.M. At work. Late getting the report done—I just couldn't focus.	You're completely hopeless. What's happened to you? You never used to be like this—you should probably retire and make way for someone who can do the job properly. Image: Frowning, forehead creased, finger waving Tone: Critical bordering on contempt	Angry 70% Exhausted 80%	I feel so deflated. Criticizing myself actually seems to add to the weight.
Thursday 2:50 P.M. Jeff's coming for therapy. I so hope he doesn't turn up.	A few years ago, I'd have been really enjoying the challenge of Jeff—how best to engage him, how to get him on board and working together. Now it seems like one big struggle. I've really lost it, I can't keep up the pace, time to put myself out to pasture. Image: Slumped body, then calm Tone: Contempt at first, then changed to a bit of warmth and understanding	Depressed 75% Exhausted 70% then some energy 50%	Fortunately, I realized after writing this that it wasn't working at all. I took myself in hand, found a bit of compassion for myself before the session, and managed to connect really well with him. Good session—but it was because I changed my tune.
Thursday 9:25 P.M. Watching TV, but thoughts just going round and round.	What am I going to do? I've really gone downhill. Doing a lousy job. Time to retire. No energy to see my friends, haven't seen Stacey for months, nor Jenny, nor Larry . . . . Image: On couch, slumped again Tone: Moderately despairing	Depressed 70% Anxious 40% Guilty 75%	Hitting myself over the head all the time with these kinds of thoughts isn't helping at all—I just feel worse.

When she reflected on the week's diary entries, Erica was struck by the frequency and intensity of her self-criticism, and she realized just how unhelpful this was for her recovery. Reviewing the week with Fatima, Erica reflected:

> What an amazing difference it made when I noticed how condemning I was of myself—I was setting myself up for failure, setting us up for an awful session. Thinking about it now, it was because I didn't want to let Jeff down that I took myself in hand and gave myself the compassion and understanding I needed. It's what I've got to do for myself, isn't it? I can't just do it when others are involved. I need to do it for myself and recognize that I'd never suggest to clients that they hammer themselves hard for every mistake they make when it's just a few months after their mother's death.

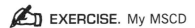 EXERCISE. My MSCD

We suggest making seven photocopies of the MSCD, one for each day. Over the next week, see if you can complete two or three entries per day. Feel free to make even more entries if you can. If it works better to do more on some days, less on others, that's fine too. The overall goal is to become mindful of your self-critical voice, notice how it operates in your life, and consider whether it's achieving results that work for you.

MY MINDFULNESS OF SELF-CRITICISM DIARY

Date/time/situation (perceived threat)	Self-critical phrase(s) I used. What was the tone of voice? Were there any images (e.g., finger pointing) or a felt sense (e.g., harshness) that accompanied the voice?	Emotions and body sensations (0–100%)	Consequences—helpful or unhelpful? How did I feel? How well did it work?

Self-Reflective Questions

How did you feel about using the MSCD? Did anything stop you? What?

_____

_____

_____

_____

_____

_____

_____

_____

_____

_____

_____

What was your experience of using it? How did that feel?

_____

_____

_____

_____

_____

_____

_____

_____

_____

_____

_____

_____

_____

Did anything about doing the diary come as a surprise? What?

_____

_____

_____

_____

_____

_____

_____

_____

_____

_____

_____

_____

_____

What have you learned from your experience that may be valuable in working with clients who are high in self-criticism?

_____

_____

_____

_____

_____

_____

_____

_____

_____

_____

_____

_____

_____

How do you think this diary would work for other aspects of the flow of compassion—for instance, how might it work if it were the Mindfulness of Criticizing Other People Diary or the Mindfulness of Feeling Criticized Diary?

_____

_____

_____

_____

_____

_____

_____

_____

_____

_____

_____

_____

_____

Midprogram Assessment

In Module 1, you completed measures of attachment avoidance and anxiety, fears of compassion, and self-compassion. You also selected and described a challenging problem to keep in mind as you work through the book. Treatment gains in therapy have been linked to the use of ongoing assessment and feedback across the course of therapy (Reese, Norsworthy, & Rowlands, 2009), and as we've reached the halfway point in the modules, let's revisit the measures and consider any movement that may have occurred, particularly in relation to the problem you identified in Module 1.

 EXERCISE. Midprogram Assessment: ECR, FOC, and CEAS-SC

First, let's revisit the items from the adapted ECR-RS, our measure of attachment avoidance and anxiety. To score it, sum your responses across the first six items to get a measure of attachment avoidance, and then sum the last three items to get a measure of attachment anxiety. As you've seen previously, the direction of the numbers changes in the middle of the measure because the first four items are reverse-scored. Just circle the response that best fits your experience and then sum up your scores.

ECR-RS: MIDPROGRAM ASSESSMENT

Please read each of the following statements and rate the extent to which you believe each statement best describes your feelings about **close relationships in general.**	Strongly disagree						Strongly agree
1. It helps to turn to people in times of need.	7	6	5	4	3	2	1
2. I usually discuss my problems and concerns with others.	7	6	5	4	3	2	1
3. I usually talk things over with people.	7	6	5	4	3	2	1
4. I find it easy to depend on others.	7	6	5	4	3	2	1
5. I don't feel comfortable opening up to others.	1	2	3	4	5	6	7
6. I prefer not to show others how I feel deep down.	1	2	3	4	5	6	7
7. I often worry that others do not really care about me.	1	2	3	4	5	6	7
8. I'm afraid that other people may abandon me.	1	2	3	4	5	6	7
9. I worry that others won't care about me as much as I care about them.	1	2	3	4	5	6	7

Attachment Avoidance (sum items 1–6):	_____
Attachment Anxiety (sum items 7–9):	_____

Now let's revisit the items from the FOCS. Take a few minutes to complete and score the following items, which assess feelings of reluctance to relate compassionately to others, receive compassion from others, and to direct compassion toward yourself. Keep in mind that the items below are just a sampling of a few items from the FOC scale, combined with a few summary items developed for this book (the full, validated scale was too long to include in this book). It hasn't been validated, so please don't use it with clients or in research—you can download the full, validated scale at *https://compassionatemind.co.uk/resources/scales.*

FOCS ITEMS: MIDPROGRAM ASSESSMENT

Please use this scale to rate the extent to which you agree with each statement.	Do not agree at all		Somewhat Agree		Completely Agree
1. Being too compassionate makes people soft and easy to take advantage of.	0	1	2	3	4
2. I fear that being too compassionate makes people an easy target.	0	1	2	3	4
3. I fear that if I am compassionate, some people will become dependent upon me.	0	1	2	3	4
4. I find myself holding back from feeling and expressing compassion toward others.	0	1	2	3	4
5. I try to keep my distance from others even if I know they are kind.	0	1	2	3	4
6. Feelings of kindness from others are somehow frightening.	0	1	2	3	4
7. When people are kind and compassionate toward me, I "put up a barrier."	0	1	2	3	4
8. I have a hard time accepting kindness and caring from others.	0	1	2	3	4
9. I worry that if I start to develop compassion for myself, I will become dependent upon it.	0	1	2	3	4
10. I fear that if I become too compassionate toward myself, I will lose my self-criticism and my flaws will show.	0	1	2	3	4
11. I fear that if I am more self-compassionate, I will become a weak person or my standards will drop.	0	1	2	3	4
12. I struggle with relating kindly and compassionately toward myself.	0	1	2	3	4

Note. This adaptation involves a limited selection of items from the FOC scale as well as additional summary items developed for this book. It was developed so that readers of this book could have a brief way of tracking their progress in working through the modules. As such, this selection of items has not been validated and is not appropriate for use in either research or clinical work. Readers can acquire a copy of the complete, validated version of the scale which is appropriate for research and clinical purposes at *https://compassionatemind.co.uk/resources/scales.*

Fears of Extending Compassion (sum items 1–4): _____
Fears of Receiving Compassion (sum items 5–8): _____
Fears of Self-Compassion (sum items 9–12): _____

Finally, let's revisit the CEAS-SC.

CEAS-SC: MIDPROGRAM ASSESSMENT

When I'm distressed or upset by things . . .	Never									Always
1. I am *motivated* to engage and work with my distress when it arises.	1	2	3	4	5	6	7	8	9	10
2. I *notice* and am *sensitive* to my distressed feelings when they arise in me.	1	2	3	4	5	6	7	8	9	10
3. I am *emotionally moved* by my distressed feelings or situations.	1	2	3	4	5	6	7	8	9	10
4. I *tolerate* the various feelings that are part of my distress.	1	2	3	4	5	6	7	8	9	10
5. I *reflect on* and *make sense* of my feelings of distress.	1	2	3	4	5	6	7	8	9	10
6. I am *accepting, noncritical,* and *nonjudgmental* of my feelings of distress.	1	2	3	4	5	6	7	8	9	10
7. I direct my *attention* to what is likely to be helpful to me.	1	2	3	4	5	6	7	8	9	10
8. I *think* about and come up with helpful ways to cope with my distress.	1	2	3	4	5	6	7	8	9	10
9. I take the *actions* and do the things that will be helpful to me.	1	2	3	4	5	6	7	8	9	10
10. I create inner feelings of *support, helpfulness,* and *encouragement*.	1	2	3	4	5	6	7	8	9	10

Compassionate Engagement (sum items 1–6): _____
Compassionate Action (sum items 7–10):   _____

Now that the measures are completed, let's revisit the challenge or problem you identified in Module 1. Before considering your challenge, let's revisit those of our three companion therapists.

EXAMPLE: Revisiting Fatima's Challenging Problem

Fatima identified her struggle with a client who both reminds her of herself at a younger age and who is sometimes hostile toward her. This has prompted feelings of self-doubt around her competency as a therapist, and feelings of wanting to avoid meeting with the client.

> **Fatima's current reflection:** Although I'm still struggling with this client, the exercises have helped me bring a more compassionate understanding to her behavior and my reactions to it. The three systems and social shaping exercises have really helped with that, as I can see how her history would shape the behaviors in her that were triggering me, in response to her own feelings of threat. It's also helped me realize how my own reactions make sense in light of my history. The safe-place imagery has helped as well, and the conversations with Erica have motivated me to reconnect with my social circles and work on being better able to accept help from people who care about me. I've still been experiencing some self-criticism and self-doubts around my challenges with my client, and I'm looking forward to the parts of the program that deal with that.

 EXAMPLE: Revisiting Joe's Challenging Problem

Having recently changed jobs, Joe now finds himself in a position with high productivity expectations, and with a supervisor he experiences as overbearing and more concerned with billable hours than with the quality of care being provided to clients. Joe has been experiencing feelings of irritability and anger around this issue, and is troubled that these feelings have "seeped out" into his personal life in his interactions with his wife and children.

> **Joe's current reflection:** My supervisor has continued the same behavior, which has continued to trigger me. When I considered my history, it made sense that he is so good at pushing my buttons. That helped me not be so neurotic about it, thinking that there must be something wrong with me. Pragmatically, the things that have helped the most have been the breathing and mindfulness exercises. I've gotten better at noticing when my threat system is activated and the breathing helps me re-center a bit, which has helped me be more present for my clients and my family.

 EXAMPLE: Revisiting Erica's Challenging Problem

Erica's choice to begin the SP/SR program was preceded by a challenging 6-month period following her mother's death. For the first couple of months following her mother's passing, Erica struggled with overwhelming grief, taking an extended time off from work, and pulling back from her social activities. Although her grief has softened over time, Erica has struggled to re-engage with her life, and hasn't really resumed the activities that fell away during her period of intense grief. Most troublingly, despite historically feeling very passionate about her work, she's noticed that her motivation has yet to return; instead, she fantasizes about retirement and experiences self-criticism around not feeling as engaged and committed to her clients as she's used to feeling.

> **Erica's current reflection:** It's been interesting to think about the three circles in relation to my problems. My main challenging emotion has been sadness, which doesn't neatly fit into the circles. But I can see that my drive system has really been underactivated since my mother died, and even though I'm not really grieving any more, I'm aware that when she died (along with my divorce 2 years ago), I lost a lot of what had helped me feel safe. I think in response to that, I've done a lot of avoidance and have generally been less invested in relationships, which were what used to excite me. The program has helped me understand how all that makes sense, and how it isn't so much my fault. That said, I need to get moving. I have some experience in behavioral activation approaches, so I know how to do that, and the co-therapy dyad work with Fatima has really helped. It's been exciting to feel helpful to her, and to feel some genuine liking passing back and forth between us.

 EXERCISE. Revisiting My Challenging Problem

Once again, set aside some time to do the exercise in a quiet, comfortable place where you'll be undisturbed, maybe with a nice cup of tea or coffee. By now, you'll probably recognize that this suggestion is aimed at helping to get your safeness system online and working for you, which will help you approach your challenge in a flexible, reflective way, rather than through the narrow lens of your threat system. So sit back, relax, spend a few moments doing some soothing rhythm breathing, and when you're ready, flip back to Module 1 and reread your description of the challenging problem you identified. After you've brought it to mind, take some time to reflect on this challenge and how you're currently experiencing it in your life. Have there been any shifts in how you understand this problem? In how it makes sense that you would struggle with it, given your history and the tricky ways our brains work? Have you noticed any shifts in how you are experiencing yourself in relation to this challenge? Consider how what you've learned about CFT may have impacted your experience of this problem, and of the version of you that has struggled with it. Have any aspects of the program been helpful? Have there been any obstacles along the way? How have you worked with them?

REVISITING MY CHALLENGING PROBLEM

💭 Self-Reflective Questions

What do you make of your midway ratings on the questionnaires? How do you feel about the changes or lack of changes? What do you notice about how you feel? How do you feel about how you feel?

_____

_____

_____

_____

_____

_____

_____

_____

_____

_____

_____

_____

_____

_____

What was your experience as you revisited your challenging situation or problem? How was it different from your reflections in Module 1?

_____

_____

_____

_____

_____

_____

_____

_____

_____

_____

_____

_____

_____

_____

Did any difficulties or obstacles come up for you as you revisited the challenging problem? If so, how do you make sense of these obstacles? Does it make sense that you would have them?

_____

_____

_____

_____

_____

_____

_____

_____

_____

_____

_____

_____

_____

_____

What lessons can you draw from your experience that might be helpful for your work with clients?

_____

_____

_____

_____

_____

_____

_____

_____

_____

_____

_____

_____

_____

_____

How does your experience of this module relate to your understanding of the CFT model and how to apply it?

_____

_____

_____

_____

_____

_____

_____

_____

_____

_____

_____

_____

_____

_____

PART II

Cultivating Compassionate Ways of Being

MODULE 18

Different Versions of the Self: The Threat-Based Self

Research in affective neuroscience has identified a number of basic evolved emotion regulation systems in humans and other animals (e.g., Panksepp & Biven, 2012; LeDoux, 1998). You may have noticed that when you're in different emotional states—happy, afraid, angry, peaceful—it may seem as if a different version of you has shown up. Many of us can find ourselves cringing when reflecting on how we've behaved when we were feeling angry or depressed, because our actions at those times were so different from how we like to think of ourselves. This can be confusing and distressing, and is often a basis for self-criticism. However, from the perspective of CFT, such experiences make perfect sense. A significant theme in CFT is that *different evolved emotions and motivations organize our minds and bodies in very different ways*, leading to very different patterns of attention, thinking and reasoning, mental imagery, felt emotional experience, motivation, and behavior (Gilbert, 2009, 2010). In CFT, this complex interaction is frequently depicted in "spider diagrams," such as the one in Figure M18.1.

In CFT, the configuration of experience produced by this complex interaction of mental processes is sometimes reflected in the language of "multiple selves": For example, we might say, "It sounds like your angry self was running the show last night." The observation that different emotions and motivational states can powerfully organize patterns of experience in us is important for developing self-compassion, because it helps us understand how we can get caught up in such confounding patterns of feeling, thinking, and behavior. CFT also discusses the concept of social mentalities: that is, interpersonal orientations grounded in basic motives (e.g., caregiving, competitive, defensive, compassionate) that organize how we experience and relate to others, and sometimes how we relate to ourselves (Gilbert, 2010). Like emotions and motives, these social mentalities can organize our experience in very different ways. Consider, for example, the

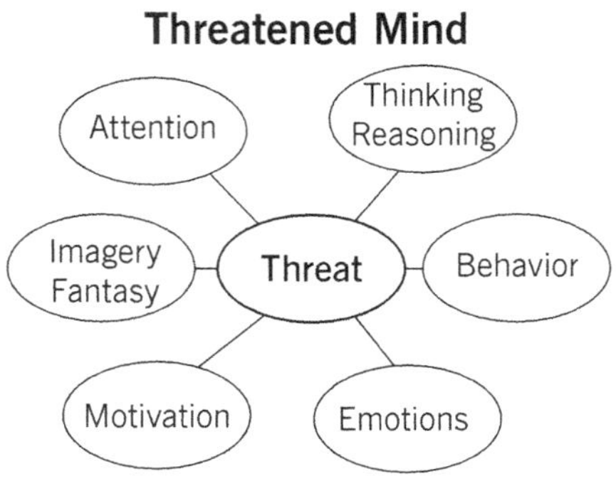

Threatened Mind

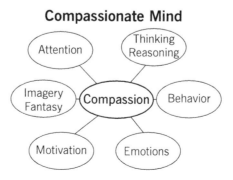

FIGURE M18.1. How threat organizes our experience. From Gilbert (2009), *The Compassionate Mind*. Reprinted with permission from Little, Brown Book Group.

differences in how you experience others, depending upon whether you are relating to them from a competitive, defensive, or caregiving perspective. Can you imagine how differently you would pay attention to others, think about them, picture them in your mind, feel about them, be motivated to treat them, and behave toward them depending upon which of these mentalities was organizing your mind and emotions?

Understanding the powerful ways such emotional and motivational states organize our minds can help clients relate more compassionately to their own struggles: "Ahh . . . so that's why I think, feel, and act that way when those emotions are triggered." It creates the possibility of having compassion for this version of the self that struggled in that difficult situation. It also gives clients, and us, a way forward. Whereas we can't choose or control the ways these different emotions, motivations, and social mentalities organize our minds, we *can* choose to purposely cultivate different motivations and ways of relating to others and ourselves. Unsurprisingly, in CFT, we focus on cultivating and strengthening *compassionate* motivations and mentalities to organize us in ways that can be particularly helpful in working effectively with suffering—our own, and that of our clients (see Figure M18.2).

Compassionate Mind

FIGURE M18.2. How compassion organizes our experience. From Gilbert (2009), *The Compassionate Mind*. Reprinted with permission from Little, Brown Book Group.

The next few modules focus on helping you explore these different perspectives. In this module, we ask you to recall a time when you experienced a sense of threat (e.g., anger, anxiety, fear) or perhaps a threat-anchored social mentality (e.g., defensiveness), and explore how that response organized your mind. Then in Module 19, you'll imagine how compassion might have organized things differently in the same situation. Let's start with an example from Joe.

 EXAMPLE: Joe's Reflection

Briefly describe the situation.

Two evenings ago, I came home from a really irritating day at work. I had just sat down with a beer, looking to relax for a bit, when Gwen came in and asked me "How was work?" in this chipper voice. I just snapped at her, "How do you think it was? It was **great**. *Just like* **every day** *at this* **wonderful job** *is* **great**. *I just can't wait to go back.* **Thanks for asking**." *I was just so nasty and sarcastic. She got quiet and avoided me the rest of the evening.*

What emotion or motivation was running the show for you? What would go in the middle of that spider diagram?

Definitely irritation, and maybe even anger. I was definitely irritated.

What emotions or bodily experience did you notice?

I was irritated, and I could feel it all over in my body. Right as she asked about my day, my body tensed up, particularly in my abdomen, neck, and forehead. My jaw clenched. I could feel that irritable energy—you know, feeling this strong motivation to snap at her even though I know that is about the worst thing I could do at that moment. And I was right; it sure didn't help. That tenseness stayed with me for the rest of the night.

Where was your attention focused during the situation? Was it broad or narrowly focused?

During the interaction, it was definitely narrowly focused on how awful my day had been, and how she must have known that, and my irritation about how she spoke to me. Later, it stayed narrowly focused, but the focus was on feeling terrible about how I'd spoken to Gwen.

Describe your thinking and reasoning during the experience. What were you thinking? Was your thinking narrowly focused, ruminative, or open and reflective?

My thinking was narrow and ruminative—I kept stewing about the same stuff over and over—that she knows I've been struggling at work and that asking how my day was just rubs it in. That she's the one who encouraged me to take that job in the first place. I was so angry. After, I kept thinking about how badly I'd handled it, about what a terrible husband I am for snapping at her when she's only trying to help and to cheer me up. I wanted to apologize, but I was afraid she'd tell me to go to hell.

What was your mental imagery like during the experience? What images or scenarios were running through your mind?

I don't know if there was any imagery going on when we were talking, but there was a lot afterward. First, I kept replaying her asking me over and over in my mind, and remembering how she had encouraged me to change jobs. Later, it was all the interaction—watching myself be nasty to her again and again in my head like a movie. I also imagined her telling me that she was through taking it, and that she was going to take the kids and move out. That was terrible. I guess I'm afraid it will come to that— that at some point, she's just going to be done with me.

What was your motivation like? What did you want to do?

Well, obviously during the situation I wanted to lash out at her, and that's what I did. After, I guess I found myself wanting to both leave the house and to apologize.

What was your behavior like? What did you do?

I've already described what I did during the situation, but after, I just hid out in my study. I sat there in my chair for the rest of the evening, zoning out on computer games, playing things out in my mind, feeling ashamed and worried. Once I knew she was in bed and probably asleep, I changed and slipped into bed as quietly as possible.

Reflecting back, how do you feel about how that experience went?

Really regretful. Things were better the next day, but that was because of Gwen. She gave me some space in the morning but was still nice and didn't seem to hold it against me. She's really better than I deserve. I never want to treat her that way.

Now let's give the exercise a try. Choose a relatively recent threat experience that may still be vivid in your mind. Considering the questions that Joe just answered, take a few moments to imagine this situation (and perhaps, as Joe did, the period afterward if that seems relevant) and the different ways your response to it played out in your mind, body, and behavior. Finally, consider how you feel looking back at this challenging situation and the experiences it triggered in you.

✍ **EXERCISE.** Exploring How Threat Organizes My Mind and Body

In this exercise, consider a recent situation that triggered a threat response or motivation in you, and then explore the way that response organized your mind.

Briefly describe the situation.

What emotion or motivation was running the show for you? What would go in the middle of that spider diagram?

What emotions or bodily experience did you notice?

Where was your attention focused during the situation? Was it broad or narrowly focused?

Describe your thinking and reasoning during the experience. What were you thinking? Was your thinking narrowly focused, ruminative, or open and reflective?

What was your mental imagery like during the experience? What images or scenarios were running through your mind?

What was your motivation like? What did you want to do?

What was your behavior like? What did you do?

Reflecting back, how do you feel about how that experience went?

☁ Self-Reflective Questions

Consider your experience of this module. What did you notice as you reflected upon the ways that your threat-based emotion or motive organized your mind? What emotions and bodily experience came up for you?

_____

_____

_____

_____

_____

_____

_____

_____

_____

_____

_____

_____

_____

Did you notice any obstacles or resistance? If so, how did you understand and work with them?

_____

_____

_____

_____

_____

_____

_____

_____

_____

_____

_____

_____

_____

_____

How useful did you find the spider diagram as a way to think about your emotions and motives?

_____

_____

_____

_____

_____

_____

_____

_____

_____

_____

_____

_____

_____

_____

Is the spider diagram something that you would consider using with clients? If so, how would you use it?

_____

_____

_____

_____

_____

_____

_____

_____

_____

_____

_____

_____

_____

Cultivating the Compassionate Self

For the rest of the book, we focus on cultivating compassionate ways of relating and working with different experiences and emotions. It's important to say that in CFT, the cultivation of compassion isn't approached as a *technique* that we *apply*, but an adaptive *way of life* that we *cultivate*. A growing body of research demonstrates that compassion meditation and compassionate ways of being in the world are associated with a host of positive outcomes, including decreased anxiety, depression, stress hormones, inflammation, and increased immune system functioning (Frederickson, Cohn, Coffee, Pek, & Finkel, 2008; Pace et al., 2009; Pace et al., 2013; Neff, Kirkpatrick, & Rude, 2007); improved empathy (Mascaro, Rilling, Negi, & Raison, 2013; Hutcherson, Seppälä, & Gross, 2015); improved emotion regulation (Lutz, Brefczynski-Lewis, Johnstone, & Davidson, 2008; Kemeny et al., 2012; Jazaieri et al., 2013; Desbordes et al., 2012); prosocial behavior (Leiberg, Limecki, & Singer, 2011); and increases in experiences of social connectedness (Hutcherson, Seppälä, & Gross, 2008), well-being (Neff, 2011), and resilience (Neff & McGehee, 2010). Benefits are also seen in the workplace, including increased organizational performance, employee productivity, and employee engagement (Cameron, Mora, Leutscher, & Calarco, 2011) (see Seppälä, 2016, for a nice summary of this literature). In this module, we introduce a practice that can serve as a framework for the cultivation of a compassionate version of the self to help you and your clients develop compassionate mental attributes that will help you (and them) work kindly and courageously with suffering and life's struggles.

The Compassionate-Self Practice:
An Acting Approach to Cultivating Compassion

In the previous module, you explored how threat-related emotions, motivations, and social mentalities can organize your experience. In this module, you'll consider how your experience can become organized by cultivating a compassionate motivation. The compassionate-self practice isn't just an isolated technique in CFT; it provides an organizing framework for all the compassionate mind-training practices that we might use with our clients.

One common obstacle for clients (and perhaps in our own self-practice) is the tendency to get so stuck in a threat-related focus that we can't imagine what a compassionate perspective might look like. Another is that we just can't imagine ourselves responding compassionately, because that is so far away from our current experience of ourselves. Given the frequency of such obstacles, CFT uses an acting approach to develop a wise, strong, and caring version of ourselves, which we call the *compassionate self*. In compassionate-self practice, the goal is to try to let go of judgments about ourselves (or the situation) regarding whether compassion might or might not be possible—or whether we feel we have the compassionate attributes involved in the practice. Instead, we follow the approach that actors use to get into a role, character, or motivation. Although actors sometimes play roles that may be quite similar—or at least familiar—to how they experience themselves, they are also often asked to portray roles that are entirely different from how they see themselves. Let's consider the skills actors use to get into various roles. Sometimes they use memories of times they've felt like the character or had experiences similar to those of the character they're playing. They might also do research or spend time imagining how this character might think, feel, or behave in various situations. Often, they will spend time observing people who have similar qualities to the role they are going to play, and from this, practice trying to embody certain qualities of the character (e.g., voice tone, facial expression, body posture, and movements).

Just like an actor playing the role of a deeply compassionate being, rather than considering if we are or are not compassionate, we imagine *what it would be like if we did possess a variety of compassionate attributes*—and how we might think, feel, pay attention, and behave from that compassionate perspective. As you work with the next exercise, don't worry if this compassionate self is different from how you typically experience yourself. The idea is to imagine what it might be like *if you did* have these qualities—how you would feel, think, be motivated to behave, and then actually behave.

If you find yourself getting caught up in distracting thoughts or struggling with resistance, see if it's possible to relate compassionately to these experiences: "It's not easy to do this. It makes sense that I would struggle while learning it. This will help me deeply understand the sorts of struggles my clients might have with this practice." Then gently bring your attention back to imagining what it might be like to have these compassionate qualities. Some people find it helpful to reconnect by starting with the body—creating a compassionate facial expression (e.g., a kind half-smile), and imagining how one's body would feel as a strong, kind, wise, compassionate being. Some CFT therapists even ask clients to get up and walk around the room in the role of their compassionate selves—imagining how they might feel, walk, and interact as this compassionate version of themselves. The key is to *find a way that works for you (and, in therapy, for each individual client)*—that enables you to imagine and begin to inhabit this compassionate perspective. Let's give it a try.

✍️ EXERCISE. The Compassionate Self Practice

In this exercise, we're going to imagine what it would be like to be a deeply compassionate person, filled with compassion, kindness, wisdom, confidence, and courage.

Let's start by preparing the body with soothing rhythm breathing. Sitting in a comfortable position with your head in an upright, dignified posture, take a minute or two to slow down the breath, spending 4–5 seconds on the inhalation and exhalation. Focus your attention on the feelings of slowing: slowing down the body, slowing down the mind.

As you allow your breath to return to a normal, comfortable rhythm, imagine that your body is filled with strength and vitality. Allow yourself to take on a kind half-smile, imagining how your face might look and how you might hold yourself as a deeply kind, wise, and confident compassionate being. Take a minute or two to enjoy holding your body in this way, imagining how you might feel, look, and even how your voice might sound as this deeply compassionate being.

Now we're going to imagine what it's like to have certain compassionate qualities.

- First, imagine what it would be like to be filled with the *caring motivation to help*—a deep desire to alleviate and prevent suffering in yourself and others, and to help you and others to have happy lives. If you'd like, you might imagine this motivation building at the level of your heart, pulsing, and gradually filling your body with light or color as you increasingly feel a deep wish to be helpful to yourself and others.

- Then, imagine that along with this caring motivation, you are filled with a deep experience of wisdom. In CFT, wisdom has a number of aspects to it. One is linked to the evolutionary model, in that the compassionate self understands that we just find ourselves here, with a body and brain that we do not choose, which give rise to the experience of various thoughts, feelings, and urges. Wisdom here also links to an understanding that we've all been shaped by things in life, many of which we had little ability to choose or control. Wisdom also brings the ability to see experiences and situations from different perspectives. When difficulties arise, your wise compassionate self is able to look deeply into them—to understand the causes and conditions that produce and maintain them. Imagine being able to think flexibly, drawing upon your life experience and intuitive wisdom as you confront the challenges in your life.

- Now, imagine that with this caring motivation and wisdom, there arises within you a deep feeling of confidence, courage, and steadfast commitment to alleviate and prevent suffering—not arrogance, but a deep knowing that *"whatever arises in my mind or in my life, I will find a way to work with this, too."* Able to trust your future compassionate self to work with whatever you may face and to seek out help when you may need it, imagine being filled with the courage to confront difficult emotions and situations and the conviction to do so—to courageously look deeply into even the obstacles that scare you, or the things you may like least about yourself.

- Take a few more moments to imagine how you might feel, think, and behave as this deeply compassionate being, filled with kindness, wisdom, courageous commitment, and compassion. What would your motivation be? What understandings might arise within you? How would your body feel? Should any difficulties, pains, or obstacles arise, see if it's possible to relate kindly and compassionately toward those as well: "Ahhh . . . this is difficult. It makes sense that it might be. From this place of compassion, how might I understand this obstacle? How might I encourage myself to keep going?"

Let's consider Joe's reflection on how the practice went for him.

 EXAMPLE: Joe's Reflection

To begin, what was your experience of the exercise like? What did you notice?

Overall, I liked it. It was hard to get into it at first, but focusing on how my body might feel helped with that. It was nice to think about what it would be like to have those qualities. I'm a long way from there now, but that sounds a lot more like the guy I'd like to be at work and particularly at home with my family.

What obstacles or resistance arose during the exercise? Were there things about the practice that you didn't like or that got in the way of it being helpful?

*Initially it felt a bit contrived . . . like, "**Ooh, now I'm going to imagine being really compassionate**." But as I followed the prompts, I was kind of able to get a sense of it. I got distracted several times and found myself a little frustrated with that, but was able to get myself back on track. The big challenge for me was that while the prompts were helpful, it felt a little vague for me—it was hard to imagine being filled with kindness, or being wise, or confident without having a situation to relate it to. Again, the focus on the body was helpful, because it gave me something a little more solid to hang on to.*

What do you think might be useful in helping you connect with this compassionate perspective and deepen it for yourself?

The biggest thing for me, I think, would be to have a situation to focus on. I think it would be useful to imagine how it would feel to apply those different qualities to a specific situation, so maybe it wouldn't feel so vague.

Following Joe's lead, take a moment to consider what the compassionate self exercise was like for you: what you liked about it, what obstacles arose, and what might be helpful to consider as you connect with this compassionate perspective in the future.

EXERCISE. Reflecting on My Compassionate-Self Practice

> **To begin, what was your experience of the exercise like? What did you notice?**
>
>
>
>
>
>
>
>
>
> **What obstacles or resistance arose during the exercise? Were there things about the practice that you didn't like or that got in the way of it being helpful?**
>
>
>
>
>
>
>
>
>
> **What do you think might be useful in helping you to connect with this compassionate perspective and deepen it for yourself?**
>
>
>
>
>
>
>
>

As we mentioned above, one goal of developing your compassionate self is to set up an organizing framework for the other compassionate skills you'll be cultivating. There's nothing magical about any one practice, and this one is no exception; the key is to repeatedly shift into this compassionate mindset again and again, gradually deepening your compassionate motivation and the ways of feeling, thinking, and behaving that go with it. By taking on this role over and over, the idea is that we'll develop the mental habits (and underlying neural architecture) that will help it feel more natural, gradually closing the gap between our compassionate selves and the way we tend to experience ourselves in our day-to-day lives.

In doing this reflection above, you likely noticed some obstacles or challenges. It's important to reflect on these and to consider ways that you can deepen your experience of the practice. We want to be focused on *process* (the process of helping ourselves create compassionate mental states in our minds) rather than technique (using the exact same words/procedures every time). So as you become more familiar with the practice and how you experience it, don't be afraid to experiment with the practice a bit as you explore and discover aspects that help you feel and think compassionately, and other bits that aren't as helpful or that may get in the way.

Self-Reflective Questions

How did you relate to this exercise? Were there any parts of yourself or internal voices that were questioning it? If so, what did they say? And what did you do with these voices?

_____

_____

_____

_____

_____

_____

_____

_____

_____

_____

_____

_____

_____

_____

Does your own experience contain any implications for how you might facilitate the compassionate self in your clients? What might you say or do that could assist people who might question the approach, or struggle to engage with the compassionate self?

_____

_____

_____

_____

_____

_____

_____

_____

_____

_____

_____

_____

_____

_____

MODULE 20

The Compassionate Self in Action

In the previous module, you practiced imagining what it would be like to be filled with various compassionate qualities. You may have noticed that Joe noted an obstacle in his reflection: that the practice felt a bit vague without a specific situation toward which the different compassionate qualities would be directed. This is a fairly common experience; it can be hard to imagine things like caring, wisdom, strength, and commitment without a situation to which these attributes are being applied. So, learning from Joe's experience, let's explore a way to make the practice more concrete—by applying it to the real-life challenges we explored in Module 18.

In this practice, you'll again connect with the mindset of the compassionate self by using the compassionate-self practice described in Module 19. Then you'll imagine how this compassionate version of you would experience and relate to the challenging problem you described in Module 18, as you engage with it from the caring, wise, courageous perspective of the compassionate self. You can take as much or as little time as you like. The key isn't the amount of time you spend so much as the felt experience of inhabiting the compassionate self in body and mind, as you imagine what it would be like to be filled with these compassionate qualities.

Let's take a look at how this exercise played out for Joe.

EXAMPLE: Joe's Practice Reflection

Briefly describe the situation.

Two evenings ago, I came home from a really irritating day at work. I had just sat down with a beer, looking to just relax for a bit, when Gwen came in and asked me "How was work?" in this chipper voice. I just snapped at her, "How do you think it was? It was **great**. *Just like* **every day** *at this* **wonderful job** *is* **great**. *I just can't wait to go back.* **Thanks for asking**." *I was just so nasty and sarcastic. She got quiet and avoided me the rest of the evening.*

See if it's possible to look back with compassion on the struggling version of you in that situation, seeing how difficult it was for you. Take a few moments, maybe engaging your soothing breathing and reengaging with the compassionate-self practice from the previous module. From this compassionate perspective of caring and understanding, how do you feel about this struggling version of yourself? What do you understand about him or her?

Huh. That's kind of a weird question. I feel bad for him, you know. He . . . I mean . . . I was just beat. I was just sitting there, trying to relax after a lousy day at work. I know that Gwen was just trying to be friendly, but I wasn't ready for that yet. I just needed some space to myself, to unwind from the day. I snapped at her—and I feel terrible about that because that's not how I want to treat her—but I didn't want to hurt her, I just wanted some space.

Knowing what you know about yourself and your previous experience, does it make sense that you reacted in the way that you did? Let's try to *understand* your reaction rather than judge it.

It does make sense. You know, despite what I just wrote, I think maybe I did want to poke at Gwen a little bit. I was angry. She was so upbeat, I felt invalidated—like she was just completely ignoring the fact that right now, my job is really hard, and most of my workdays are pretty miserable. So it felt pretty crappy to have her approach me like that, even though I know she meant well and was just trying to lift my spirits. That must be hard for her, too, because it's like she can't win—if she's upbeat, I get mad, and if she's down about it like I am, she might worry that it makes it worse. I know she feels guilty about encouraging me to go for this new job, even though it wasn't her fault that it hasn't turned out the way we hoped it would.

Now let's imagine that spider diagram again, this time putting compassion right in the middle. See if it's possible to imagine what it would be like to be back in that situation again, this time as your caring, wise, courageously compassionate self. Imagine being back in that situation, this time experiencing it through the mindset of this deeply compassionate perspective. Try to imagine this (and even to write it down) as if it were happening again, in real time. From this compassionate mindset, what do you feel? How do these feelings play out in your body?

I feel calm. Not totally relaxed, because it was a difficult day, but calm . . . like, sort of peaceful even though the day hadn't gone as I'd hoped.

From this compassionate mindset, where is your attention focused during the situation? Is it broadly or narrowly focused?

Definitely more broadly focused than it was. Rather than being focused on the crappy day or on being irritated at what Gwen said, my compassionate self is paying attention to how nice it is to be home and to be with her. I'm aware of the many things in my life that are actually really good, even though my job isn't the best right now. Like how she is just trying to cheer me up. And how smart and beautiful she is, and how much I appreciate her. And how I'm lucky to have a family that loves me and stands by me. I'm crying just thinking about them. I love them so much. I just want them to know that.

From this compassionate mindset, what are you thinking about during the experience? How are you making sense of it?

I think I got in a lot of the thoughts in that previous question. As I mentioned, my compassionate self has a much broader and more flexible perspective. I'm able to see things from Gwen's perspective, which really was about trying to help me. That's really helpful to notice.

From this compassionate mindset, what is your motivation in this situation? What does this compassionate version of you want to do?

My compassionate self wants to help make things better for me—to do something other than just sit there and stew—and to connect with Gwen rather than push her away.

In this situation, feeling and acting from this kind, wise, compassionate mindset, what does this compassionate version of you do?

First, I don't grab a beer and sit down to stew about things—I would do something I enjoy, like go for a walk or play my guitar. Then, when Gwen gets home, instead of clinging to what I am unhappy about, I would greet her warmly and let her know how happy I am to see her, and how lucky I feel to be with her, even though things aren't easy at work right now. I'm imagining myself rubbing her shoulders and back. She loves that, and it creates closeness between us rather than the distance that came out of my snapping at her. The evening would play out really differently.

Looking back on that imagined scenario of how you might have handled things from this compassionate mindset, how do you feel?

A bit regretful and sad, imagining how differently things could have played out had I reacted differently. But also hopeful, because now instead of feeling trapped in how I was feeling, it's clear that the situation changes entirely when I show up as my compassionate self—that would really change how my time with my family went. I may never love this job, but I don't have to hate my life. I'm also looking forward to seeing my family this evening and getting a chance to show them how much I appreciate them.

> **One last question: Imagine that this caring, wise, compassionate version of you were able to go back, invisibly, to that situation and offer support, encouragement, and advice to the struggling version of you that was having such a hard time. How might you support, encourage, or advise that struggling version of you so that you could be at your best as you dealt with this challenge?**
>
> *That's easy. I'd let myself know that it makes sense that I'm having a bad day, because my job sucks right now. But I'd remind myself that there's a whole lot more to my life than that crappy job. And I'd remind myself that in a few minutes, there's a wonderful woman that I love more than anything who is going to walk through that door, and that I can either connect with her and have a fun evening with the people I love, or push her away and spend the rest of the night stewing over something I can't fix right now. I think that even when I was in a bad mood, that would be a fairly easy choice.*

Now that Joe has given us an example of how this exercise can go, let's apply the compassionate-self practice to a challenging situation in your life—perhaps the situation you described in the Module 18. You'll begin by connecting with the compassionate-self practice in the manner we did in Module 19, and then work through the reflections that follow. Remember, the key is to imagine what it would be like to relate to this challenging situation (and to the version of you that struggled in this situation) from the perspective of a caring, wise, courageously compassionate version of you. If it seems difficult, try to remind yourself that you don't have to feel like you have these qualities yet—you're just imagining what it would be like *if you did have them*, like an actor taking on a role. If any difficulties arise, see if you can extend compassion to the fact that doing this can be really challenging—imagine how you might relate to those difficulties from the perspective of your compassionate self, and what might help encourage you to keep going, even when it gets hard.

🖎 EXERCISE. My Compassionate Self in Action

Going back through the compassionate-self practice in Module 19, connect with the perspective of your compassionate self, taking as much or as little time as you like. Imagine what it would be like to be filled with these compassionate qualities: the kind, caring motivation to help; the wisdom to look deeply into suffering and understand it; and the courage to face challenges and discomfort head on and work with them. The key isn't the amount of time you spend, but the experience of inhabiting this compassionate mindset, imagining what it would be like to be filled with these compassionate qualities. Once you've done this, let's once again visit that challenging situation you described in Module 18. This time, however, try to imagine how you might have engaged with this experience from the caring, wise, courageous perspective of the compassionate self.

Briefly describe the situation.

See if it's possible to look back with compassion on the struggling version of you in that situation, seeing how difficult it was for you. Take a few moments, maybe engaging your soothing breathing and reengaging with the compassionate-self practice from the previous module. From this compassionate perspective of kindness and understanding, how do you feel about this struggling version of yourself? What do you understand about him or her?

Knowing what you know about yourself and your previous experience, does it make sense that you reacted in the way that you did? Let's try to *understand* your reaction rather than judge it.

Now let's imagine that spider diagram again, this time putting compassion right in the middle. See if it's possible to imagine what it would be like to be back in that situation again, this time as your caring, wise, courageously compassionate self. Imagine being back in that situation, this time experiencing it through the mindset of this deeply compassionate perspective. Try to imagine this (and even to write it down) as if it were happening again, in real time. From this compassionate mindset, what do you feel? How do these feelings play out in your body?

From this compassionate mindset, where is your attention focused during the situation? Is it broadly or narrowly focused?

From this compassionate mindset, what are you thinking about during the situation? How are you making sense of it?

From this compassionate mindset, what is your motivation in this situation? What does this compassionate version of you want to do?

Imagine that you are back in this situation, feeling and acting from this kind, wise, compassionate mindset. What does this compassionate version of you do?

Looking back on that imagined scenario of how you might have handled things from this compassionate mindset, how do you feel?

One last question: Imagine that this caring, wise, compassionate version of you were able to invisibly go back to that situation and offer support, encouragement, and advice to the struggling version of you that was having such a hard time in that situation. How might you support, encourage, or advise that struggling version of you so that you could be at your best as you dealt with this challenge?

Self-Reflective Questions

Comparing your experience of the compassionate self in this module with your experience of the compassionate self in the previous module, what difference (if any) did it make having a specific situation on which to focus?

_____

_____

_____

_____

_____

_____

_____

_____

_____

_____

_____

_____

_____

What obstacles or resistance arose during the exercise? Were there things about the practice that you didn't like or that got in the way of it being helpful? If so, how did you work with them, or what do you think might be helpful in working with them in the future?

_____

_____

_____

_____

_____

_____

_____

_____

_____

_____

_____

_____

Reflecting on your experience of this module, does anything stand out that might inform how you approach this process with your clients? Perhaps think of one specific client—how might your experience affect your approach with him or her?

_____

_____

_____

_____

_____

_____

_____

_____

_____

_____

_____

_____

_____

_____

MODULE 21

Deepening the Compassionate Self

In Module 15, we explored a working definition of compassion as involving both a *sensitivity* to suffering and struggle and a *commitment* to work to alleviate and prevent this suffering. In Module 19, we introduced the compassionate-self practice to help you and your clients bring this definition alive and embody compassion in your lives. Looking more closely at this definition of compassion, we see that two sets of capacities are involved: how we respond to or *engage* with suffering, and what we then *do about it*—how we prepare ourselves to alleviate and prevent suffering. CFT founder Paul Gilbert refers to these as the two *psychologies of compassion,* and in CFT, each aspect of compassion is further operationalized into the processes involved when compassion is manifested in the real world (Gilbert, 2009, 2010).

Engagement: Exploring the First Psychology of Compassion

First and perhaps foremost, compassion will require our clients to change how they relate to their suffering. Many of them will have previously coped with painful experiences and emotions by seeking to avoid or suppress them, and sometimes by attacking themselves for experiencing the suffering (which could be seen as even another nuanced method of avoidance). In helping clients develop compassion, we're working to assist them in turning *toward* their suffering with caring, wisdom, and courage. As therapists, we can sometimes observe these tendencies in ourselves as well. In this section, we explore the various attributes involved in this ability to compassionately engage with suffering, as noted in Figure M21.1 (on page 203).

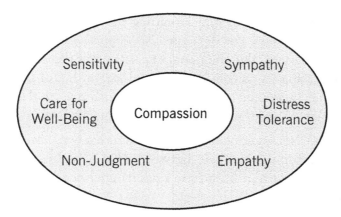

FIGURE M21.1. The first psychology of compassion: Engagement. Adapted from Gilbert (2009), *The Compassionate Mind.* Reprinted with permission from Little, Brown Book Group.

Let's briefly explore each of these qualities in a bit more detail.

• *Care for well-being.* An important starting point for compassion is a *caring motivation:* that is, experiencing a basic desire to reduce suffering and enhance the well-being and happiness of ourselves and those with whom we come into contact.

• *Sensitivity.* Sensitivity to distress involves *noticing*—becoming aware of distress and suffering—and paying attention to it, rather than blocking it out or turning away from it. With sensitivity, suffering shows up on our radar, allowing us to tune in to the person in need of care—including ourselves.

• *Sympathy.* Sympathy involves being *emotionally moved* by the experiences and feelings that we or others face. Sympathy is about *felt experience* rather than concepts or a mental understanding. For many people who are in emotional pain, feeling sympathy may be difficult; they may feel quite numb, shut off, or have learned to quickly block out feelings that arise in response to their own or others' pain. In the context of compassionate action, it's important to note that sympathy is seen as helping motivate us to approach and address suffering. However, it's important that it is not so strongly held as to get in the way of helping (e.g., by shifting the focus from the person who suffers to our own sympathetic distress).

• *Distress tolerance.* Engaging with suffering will bring us into contact with a lot of pain and discomfort, which has the potential to overwhelm us and shut off our compassion. For this reason, a core quality of compassion is distress tolerance: the ability to engage with, tolerate, and take an accepting stance toward the difficulties and discomfort that arise as we work with difficult experiences. This doesn't mean passively resigning ourselves to our pain or continuing to expose ourselves to ongoing harm; it means that we can compassionately tolerate uncomfortable experiences as we work to address them.

• *Empathy.* Empathy involves understanding the experience of the person who is suffering, whether it is ourselves or someone else. Empathy includes both an *emotional* component—resonating with the emotional experience of the person who suffers—as well as the cognitive capacity to consider and *understand* her or his experience (and if we want to go further by adding validation, how it *makes sense* that she or he may be having this experience). Empathy can easily become blocked when we feel threatened.

• *Non-judgment.* Non-judgment doesn't mean that we have no preferences or choices, or that we fail to discriminate between what is and is not helpful. Rather, it means that we try our best to refrain from criticizing or condemning our own experience or that of others.

In the next section, you'll consider two questions: *How do you feel about your ability to engage with these aspects of compassionate engagement?* and *What might you do to further cultivate these abilities?* Before considering your own experience, let's look at how Erica and Fatima explored these areas in their limited co-therapy session.

 EXAMPLE: Exploring Compassionate Engagement

FATIMA: Erica, in this module we'll be going through the six aspects of compassionate engagement from the manual, and I'll be asking you first about how you are able to experience each of the qualities, and then about what might be helpful as you develop the qualities further. Does that sound all right?

ERICA: (*Nods.*) Sounds good.

FATIMA: We'll just work our way around the circle, then. Could you talk about your experience of compassionate motivation—that is, your experience of caring for the well-being of yourself and others?

ERICA: I've always had a lot of motivation to help other people; it's given me a real sense of purpose in my life. But for a while right after Mom died, it felt like I just didn't have any motivation. I think I tried to avoid other peoples' pain so that it didn't retrigger my own. I also had a period when I didn't care much about my own well-being either—I just felt completely overwhelmed. Slowly, that caring has started to come back, and I've found myself engaging more and more with clients and other people. I've really enjoyed these meetings with you, for example. Through the practices, I'm also learning that I need to work on bringing that same warmth to myself, and to being more open to receiving help from others.

FATIMA: I'm really glad to hear that you're feeling more engaged as the grief has softened. It sounds like you've figured out some ways that you want to grow in this area. What might help you to build that caring motivation in the ways you mentioned?

ERICA: Honestly, I think I just need to find ways to keep it present in my mind, to remind myself that I want to relate kindly to myself and others. There are all sorts of therapy tools I've used to help my clients remember things like this. We talked about journaling in a previous session, and I think keeping a compassion journal that I just write a bit in every day—so it becomes a part of my routine—I think that would really help.

FATIMA: That sounds like a great idea! I should try that, too. Let's move on to the next quality: sensitivity. How well are you able to notice when you or others are suffering or struggling?

ERICA: That really depends. For myself, I'm getting better at noticing when I'm distressed, but during that period of really intense grief, there wasn't much awareness there at all—I was just *in it,* like that's just the way it was. I'm getting better at noticing those feelings coming up, and the mindfulness exercises we've done have helped with that.

FATIMA: How about noticing when other people are suffering?

ERICA: I've always been good at that—noticing shifts in people's faces or tone of voice that signaled they were feeling something. I struggled with that right after my mother died because I was so caught up in my own feelings, but generally that's something I'm pretty good at.

FATIMA: What might be helpful in developing your sensitivity even further?

ERICA: Two things come to mind. The first thing is to manage my own distress a bit better so it doesn't get in the way. It really resonated with me when we learned about the threat system and how it narrows our attention. I also want to keep practicing the mindfulness exercises, because those have seemed to give me some distance to notice what I'm experiencing rather than getting completely caught up in it.

FATIMA: That's great. I really appreciate how closely you're looking at your experience. How are you feeling?

ERICA: Really good, actually. You've definitely become one of my "safe people." (*Smiles.*)

FATIMA: (*Smiles warmly.*) Thanks. That feels really good to hear. Ready for the next area?

ERICA: Why not?

FATIMA: How about sympathy? How is that for you?

ERICA: I haven't always been the most easily moved—I'm not always crying at movies or things like that, but I definitely feel for people when I see them suffer. With my clients, I feel that in my career, I've had a decent balance between feeling for them and not being overwhelmed by their suffering—which feels important. Like I mentioned earlier, I was pretty disconnected right after my mother died, but that's been getting better.

FATIMA: How about for yourself? Are you able to feel sympathy for yourself when you're suffering or struggling?

ERICA: That's been different. Honestly, I don't know that it has ever occurred to me that I could have sympathy for *myself*. In the past, I've tended to pay very little attention to my own distress, or sometimes I just poo-poo it and expect myself to buck up and get on with things. The compassionate self exercise we did in the last module really shifted that for me, I think. When I looked back at myself struggling after my mother died, it became clear how much I was hurting then—I felt really moved by it, actually. I've had a couple of good cries since that exercise, and I think it really helped. It's the first time I've acknowledged how hard that was for me, and just let myself feel something about it. (*becoming tearful*)

FATIMA: (*Pauses, smiling gently, slightly tearful herself.*) What might help you keep growing that sympathy for yourself?

ERICA: (*Pauses.*) I think just slowing down and being willing to acknowledge when I'm hurting, and reminding myself that my pain is as valid as everyone else's. (*still tearful*)

FATIMA: (*warmly*) It is, you know. Your pain *is* as valid as everyone else's.

ERICA: (*Smiles gently, openly crying, blows nose.*) You really got me there. But you're right. It is. And I need to remember that.

FATIMA: (*Leans in, smiles.*) Ready for the next one?

ERICA: (*Smiles.*) Yeah.

FATIMA: How about distress tolerance? Are you able to cope with distress when you see it in your clients or yourself?

ERICA: I've always been pretty good at tolerating my clients' distress. I think you have to learn to do that if you're going to do this therapy thing for very long. Over my life, as I've told you, I was pretty good at managing my own as well—but I sort of fell apart in that regard after my mother died. The sadness just felt so overwhelming. Like I said, that's been gradually getting better.

FATIMA: Any ideas about how to grow that ability to tolerate distress even further?

ERICA: Really, to just use what I know, and the things I've learned recently that have been helpful, such as the soothing rhythm breathing and some of the imagery exercises. Like we do with our clients: to think about what has been helpful to me in working with distress in the past and to make sure I use it. That's what I didn't do after my mother died. The other thing would be to make sure to connect with my friends sooner rather than later. When I'm hurting, it's the last thing I feel like doing, but it also really helps.

FATIMA: (*Nods.*) Yeah, I can relate to that.

ERICA: (*Smiles.*) I thought you probably could.

FATIMA: How about empathy? Are you good at recognizing and understanding the emotions and experiences that you and others feel?

ERICA: When I'm not in threat myself, I'm good at feeling empathy for my clients. I've always felt pretty good at considering their experiences and what it might be like for them to face different situations. I haven't done as much of that for myself, mostly because I don't think I've slowed down to ask, "What am I feeling?" The mindfulness practices and just trying to remember to check in and consider what I'm feeling seem to be helping with that.

FATIMA: That's great. Anything else that might help with that?

ERICA: Maybe some journaling. Getting my feelings down on paper seems to help me look at them more objectively and see how they make sense.

FATIMA: (*Nods.*) We're on the last one, which is non-judgment. It seems like this one is about refraining from being critical when you see your clients or yourself struggling or suffering. How are you with that?

ERICA: I've never really been too judgmental of others. I mean, some people will push my buttons, but even then . . . growing up, my mother brought me up not to judge. She always said you never know the story of how people got to be the way they are. (*Pauses.*) I've gone through periods of being self-critical, though. I can treat myself quite harshly if I feel like I'm screwing up or not doing things the way I'd like.

FATIMA: What do you think might help with that?

ERICA: Really, what we were talking about before. Just giving myself permission to struggle. Because *of course* I will struggle, just like everyone else will. If I can remember that, I think it will really help.

FATIMA: (*Smiles and nods.*) That's great, Erica. That resonates with me, too. We're at the end of the exercise. Anything else you'd like to mention?

ERICA: No, but I wanted to thank you. This was really helpful for me. (*Smiles gently.*)

FATIMA: Thanks. And thank you as well. (*Smiles warmly.*)

Now it's time for you to consider the same questions: How do you experience the different qualities of compassionate engagement, and what might be helpful in assisting you to deepen these qualities? If you're doing this exercise individually, create a comfortable physical and psychological space, as you have done for previous exercises. On the other hand, if you're working with a group or a limited co-therapy pair, this might be a good exercise to explore interactively with a partner, as Erica and Fatima demonstrated.

 EXERCISE. Exploring My Compassionate Engagement

Create a comfortable setting for yourself and engage your soothing rhythm breathing. Then reflect on these different aspects of compassionate engagement.

Compassionate motivation: Explore your experience of connecting with the kind desire to help yourself and others in the face of suffering or struggle. Is this something that comes easily or is it challenging for you?

What might be helpful in further developing your compassionate motivation?

Sensitivity: Explore your experience of being able to notice and be aware of suffering and struggle when it is present in yourself or others. Is this something that comes easily or is it challenging for you?

What might be helpful in further developing your ability to compassionately notice and become aware of suffering and struggle in yourself and others?

Sympathy: Explore your experience of being moved by your observations of suffering and struggle in yourself and others. Is this something that comes easily or is it challenging for you?

What might be helpful in further developing your ability to be compassionately moved by your observations of suffering and struggle in yourself and others?

Distress tolerance: Explore your experience of being able to cope in the face of discomfort or distress without having to avoid or escape the experience. Is this something that comes easily for you or is it more challenging?

What might be helpful in further developing your ability to compassionately tolerate distress and work with it without having to avoid or escape the experience?

Empathy: Explore your experience of being able to recognize and understand the emotions that you and others are experiencing during times of suffering and struggle. Is this something that comes easily or is it challenging for you?

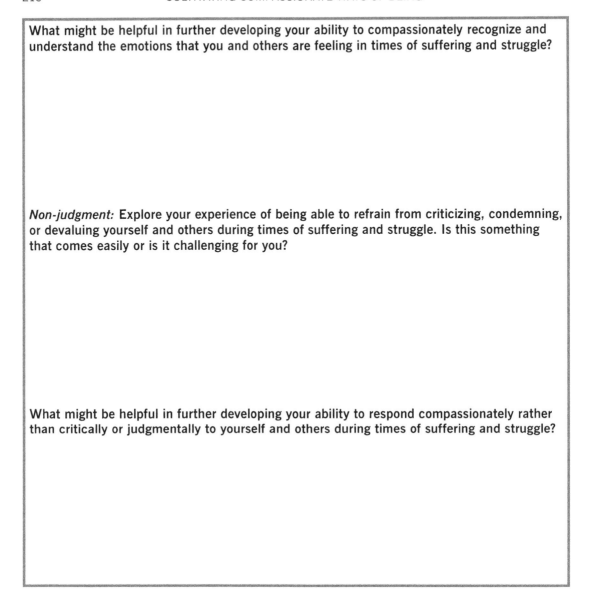

What might be helpful in further developing your ability to compassionately recognize and understand the emotions that you and others are feeling in times of suffering and struggle?

Non-judgment: **Explore your experience of being able to refrain from criticizing, condemning, or devaluing yourself and others during times of suffering and struggle. Is this something that comes easily or is it challenging for you?**

What might be helpful in further developing your ability to respond compassionately rather than critically or judgmentally to yourself and others during times of suffering and struggle?

In this module, we've focused upon exploring the first psychology of compassion: your ability to engage with suffering in compassionate ways. The second psychology of compassion involves the ways we prepare ourselves to *respond compassionately* to suffering and to do something to alleviate and prevent it. In CFT, this compassionate response is operationalized in terms of multimodal skills training that involves working with our attention, imagery, thinking and reasoning, feeling states, sensory focusing, and behavior, as noted in Figure M21.2 (on page 211). Space precludes an extended exploration of these functions in this module—but there's no need, as you'll see many of these training methods demonstrated throughout the workbook.

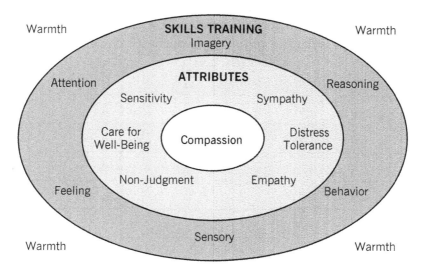

FIGURE M21.2. Compassionate attributes and skills training. Adapted from Gilbert (2009), *The Compassionate Mind.* Reprinted with permission from Little, Brown Book Group.

Self-Reflective Questions

How easy or difficult was it for you to experience the six attributes of compassionate engagement? Were some easier than others? Which?

_____

_____

_____

_____

_____

_____

_____

_____

_____

_____

_____

_____

_____

What sense do you make of your strengths and weaknesses in experiencing the six attributes? Can you track these back to earlier experiences in your life? Is it helpful to do so?

_____

_____

_____

_____

_____

_____

_____

_____

_____

_____

_____

_____

How does your experience of this module affect what you might do with clients? What strategies might you use to facilitate the six attributes in them?

_____

_____

_____

_____

_____

_____

_____

_____

_____

_____

_____

_____

_____

The six attributes of engagement and the six skills are part of the fabric of CFT. How valuable do you find this conceptualization? Is there anything you might add or change as a result of your experience?

_____

_____

_____

_____

_____

_____

_____

_____

_____

_____

_____

_____

_____

MODULE 22

Behavioral Experiments in CFT

Although to date, there is no CFT-specific research examining the effectiveness of behavioral experiments, researchers in the CBT tradition have suggested that behavioral experiments are one of the most effective strategies for therapeutic change (Bennett-Levy et al., 2004; McMillan & Lee, 2010; Salkovskis, Hackmann, Wells, Gelder, & Clark, 2007). Given these recommendations and the observation that throughout his writings, Paul Gilbert has noted that behavioral experiments can be readily adapted for CFT (Gilbert, 2010), we thought it would be useful to include a module demonstrating how behavioral experiments can be used within a CFT context.

Behavioral experiments usually start with the therapist and client identifying an idea or thought that is an obstacle to progress and is amenable to testing in the real world. Clients then rate their belief in the idea(s) on a 0–100% scale. We suggest using two kinds of rating: a *gut* or *heart level* belief and a *rational* belief, as there is often a discrepancy between how we feel "in our gut" or heart, and what we think rationally (Bennett-Levy et al., 2015; Stott, 2007; Teasdale, 1996). Then the client and therapist work together to develop an experiment that tests the validity of the two ideas/beliefs, which can occur in session or in the client's daily life. It may involve a role-play behavioral experiment in a therapy session (e.g., the therapist asks, "How about I role-play your critical voice, and you notice what you feel and what goes through your mind?"). It may involve actions taken in the outside world (e.g., "What difference does it make if I engage with my compassionate self at work?"). Another variant of behavioral experiments involves observing others (e.g., "How do other people treat themselves when they make mistakes? How well does this work for them?"). Behavioral experiments may arise spontaneously (e.g., in session, the therapist asks, "How do you think I am feeling about what you've just revealed about yourself?"). And sometimes the therapist and client set up "discovery" experiments in which the client has no idea what might happen if he or she changes his or her behavior ("How about we see whether anything changes if you practice soothing rhythm breathing for a week?"). A particular feature of behavioral experiments in CFT is that they are likely to involve exploration of the impact of different motivational systems (e.g., threat protection, compassionate self).

Sometimes a behavioral experiment can be set up around testing an old unhelpful idea (Hypothesis A) derived from a threat protection strategy (e.g., "Being really hard on myself is the best way to up my game."). Sometimes the old idea is compared with a new idea derived from the compassionate self (Hypothesis A vs. Hypothesis B) (e.g., "If I treat myself with care and compassion, just like I'd do with my son, it may be a better way to up my game."). And sometimes, an experiment is developed with the primary purpose of building evidence for a new idea, Hypothesis B (e.g., "Building my compassionate self should lead to better results."). In each of these examples, the tone is one of curious exploration: "Let's see what happens if we try this."

After designing an experiment (but before carrying it out), the participant makes predictions about what may happen. Then the participant carries out the experiment. After the experiment, the participant records his or her observations about what actually did happen, rates his or her belief in the idea(s) again, and reflects on the implications of the experience for his or her ideas about the value of compassion in his or her life. For a more in-depth treatment of behavioral experiments, see Bennett-Levy et al. (2004, 2015).

 EXAMPLE: Setting Up a Behavioral Experiment

ERICA: In this module we're going to look at how to set up and complete a behavioral experiment. How are you feeling about this one?

FATIMA: I feel a bit anxious. I've heard about these but never used them in therapy before.

ERICA: (*Smiles gently.*) I can appreciate that—it can be quite anxiety-provoking doing new things for the first time. Let's take it step by step and see how it goes.

FATIMA: (*Smiles.*) Sounds like a plan.

ERICA: To start with, can you think of an idea—maybe one you've had for quite some time—that reflects how your threat system can be an obstacle to working with your clients in the way you'd like?

FATIMA: As we've touched on already, I sometimes get caught up thinking that if I don't work long hours, I'll let my clients down.

ERICA: That one shows up for me as well. (*Smiles.*) At your gut level, how much do you believe in that idea on a 0–100% scale?

FATIMA: I suppose it's around 80%—it feels quite powerful.

ERICA: What about on a more rational, cognitive level?

FATIMA: That's a bit less, I think. Part of me knows it might not be quite true. So maybe 50%.

ERICA: Nicely done. Next, we'll tap into another perspective—Hypothesis B. To do this, it would probably be helpful for you to get in touch with your compassionate self. Shall we spend a couple of minutes doing that?

FATIMA: Sounds good.

ERICA: (*Leads Fatima through connecting with her posture and breathing, and then guides her through a brief compassionate-self practice.*) Fatima, now that you're connected with your compassionate self—the part of you that is wise, strong, and committed to your well-being—how do you see this situation? Take a few moments to think about how your compassionate self might understand and approach this issue.

FATIMA: (*Sits quietly for a few minutes, looking thoughtful.*) I'm a bit surprised, as that was easier than I thought it would be. My compassionate self recognizes that if I do a better job of taking care of myself, I'm likely to become a better therapist for my clients—which is also what my threatened self wants. It's just coming at it from a different perspective.

ERICA: (*Smiles warmly.*) Well done! OK, how strong do you rate the perspective of the compassionate self?

FATIMA: Um, I guess on the emotional, gut level, I'd say 30%. Rationally, I think it's around 50%.

ERICA: Nicely done, Fatima. You're definitely getting the hang of this. Let's see how we might test this out. What could you do over the next couple of weeks?

FATIMA: Well, it seems like I need to test both hypotheses. Maybe I should just start by sticking with what I normally do at work over the next week and see how that leaves me feeling?

ERICA: Great. That sounds good for next week. What would you think about testing out something different in the second week—a way of being at work based on the perspective of your compassionate self? How might you do that?

FATIMA: It would make sense to leave at 5:00 P.M. like everyone else does.

ERICA: That sounds like a good plan. How are you feeling about this? What predictions do you have about how it might go?

FATIMA: I think there are different answers to that question. I'm really connecting with how differently my threat-based mind and my compassionate mind see things. My threat-based mind is really anxious about changing things—worried about letting my clients down, and feeling I'm not good enough as a therapist and as a person. I know what happens next—I struggle to sleep and get caught up in self-criticism and rumination, especially at night.

ERICA: (*Warmly.*) Sounds like you've had a lot of practice getting into your threat system.

FATIMA: (*Smiles.*) I sure have! (*Pauses, thinking.*) I'm beginning to notice how good I am at slipping into that threat-filled place. Having said that, I'm getting more comfortable slowing down and reconnecting with my compassionate self. With all the practice we're doing, it's becoming clearer to me.

ERICA: What does your compassionate self think about all this?

FATIMA: (*Pauses, thinking.*) My compassionate self is telling me that although I'll feel anxious, I'm strong enough to tolerate those feelings, and that I'm likely to feel relieved—like a weight off my shoulders. Although it's understandable to want to help my clients, I'm not doing them any favors by squeezing them in at the end of an already long day.

ERICA: Well done, Fatima. I can really hear your compassionate self coming through here. Is there anything else she would hold in mind while doing this experiment?

FATIMA: She's reminding me that I can reconnect with this compassionate perspective to help manage any difficulties I experience during that second week. It's strange; it feels really grounding to know that.

Fatima continued to outline the experiment with Erica, and selected some measures to help her to observe any changes between Hypotheses A and B. She made one set of predictions about what was likely to happen based on Hypothesis A, and another set based on Hypothesis B. She then carried out the experiment, making notes on the outcomes of the first and second weeks. In particular, to help her follow through with her plan of leaving work at 5:00 P.M. each day, she made sure to practice connecting with her compassionate self each morning before starting work and grounding herself in her compassionate intention for the day (to take care of her own well-being and to tolerate threat-based feelings that might make it hard for her to leave work at 5:00). After completing the second week, she and Erica reviewed the results of the experiment (considering differences in both the self-report measures and her own reflections of the experience).

Developing Your Behavioral Experiment

Once you have absorbed the process of Fatima's experiment, have a go at developing a behavioral experiment to test out some of your less self-compassionate ideas and comparing them with ideas generated by your compassionate self. Following Fatima's example, record your ideas to be tested, your initial gut-level and rational belief ratings, set up your experiment, find some good ways to measure any progress, and make predictions about the likely outcome. Then over the next week or two, carry out the experiment, find some good ways to measure any progress, and at the end of the week, again rate your degree of belief in your original ideas, as in Fatima's example on page 218. Use the blank Behavioral Experiment Record Sheet on page 219 as a guide to help yourself with this, and try not to worry about getting it all exactly right, especially if this is the first time you've set up a behavioral experiment.

FATIMA'S BEHAVIORAL EXPERIMENT RECORD SHEET

Date	Thought/idea	Experiment	Prediction(s)	Outcome	What I learned
	What thought, idea, assumption, or belief are you testing? Is there an alternative perspective? Rate your belief in the cognition (0–100%).	Design an experiment to test the thought (e.g., test out your fears of compassion, face a situation you would otherwise avoid, drop your precautions, behave in a new way).	What do you predict will happen?	What actually happened? What did you observe? How does the outcome fit with your predictions?	What does this outcome mean for your original idea/belief? How much do you now believe it (0–100%)? Does it need to be modified? How?
9/2–9/16	Hypothesis A: If I don't meet my clients' needs for appointments by working consistently late hours, it shows a lack of care and compassion (even if the cost is exhaustion). I'd feel bad. Gut-level belief: 80% Rational belief: 50% vs. Hypothesis B: If I look after myself better, I'll feel much better in myself and be a better therapist. Gut-level belief: 30% Rational belief: 50%	Work as normal next week. In the following week go home every day at 5 P.M. Compare how I score on the following measures: • Depression, Anxiety and Stress Scale (DASS) • Brief Irritability Scale • Compassion for Self and Others scale • Self-rating of quality of each therapy session (0–10)	I'm not sure. My "threatened mind" says that I'll feel incredibly guilty at having to put people off. This will cause me quite a lot of anxiety, and make me ruminate at night. I may feel quite irritable. My therapy may not be quite as good if I'm seeing a lot more people, but I'll feel better about it. vs. My compassionate mind says looking after myself will feel like such a relief. I may actually get time in the evenings to go to yoga—or even go to an early-evening movie with Robin! I suspect my therapy will be much more enjoyable and probably a whole lot better. And in reality, will waiting a day or so more be so bad for my clients?	As usual, I was pretty exhausted in the first week. I felt irritable and exhausted at home on 4/5 nights. Ratings on the DASS and on the irritability scales were concerning :(. And I realized from the ratings that the quality of my therapy started to decline in the afternoon, so I actually felt dissatisfied with an average of 3 sessions a day. In week 2, it was such a sense of liberation to be able to leave work at 5 P.M.! On the first couple of days I felt a bit guilty, but by the 4th day, I realized from the ratings that my energy and compassion were so much greater than in the first week, and my scores on the two scales were lower. I averaged only 0.8 dissatisfying sessions in the compassion week.	Rerating of thoughts: "Not responding to clients' needs shows a lack of care and compassion." Gut-level belief: 30% Rational belief: 20% "If I look after myself better, I'll feel much better in myself and I'll be a better therapist." Gut-level belief: 80% Rational belief: 80% On all the measures, the benefits of looking after myself better far outweighed the costs. Once I was over the initial guilt, I felt so much better in myself. And my therapy was so much better, as my self-ratings of quality showed.

218

MY BEHAVIORAL EXPERIMENTS RECORD SHEET

Date	Thought/idea	Experiment	Prediction(s)	Outcome	What I learned
	What thought, idea, assumption, or belief are you testing? Is there an alternative perspective? Rate your belief in the cognition (0–100%).	Design an experiment to test the thought (e.g., test out your fears of compassion, face a situation you would otherwise avoid, drop your precautions, behave in a new way).	What do you predict will happen?	What actually happened? What did you observe? How does the outcome fit with your predictions?	What does this outcome mean for your original idea/belief? How much do you now believe it (0–100%)? Does it need to be modified? How?

Remember, the key to this process is how you use the compassionate self to help generate Hypothesis B, develop the experiment, and come up with predictions of what will happen. It may be helpful to shift into the mindset of your compassionate self before trying the alternative behavior, to help you maintain your motivation and tolerate any experiences of threat that arise. Finally, this compassionate mindset will be helpful as you reflect upon the experiment; if your reflection is driven by your threat-based or self-critical mind, it may be difficult to reflect clearly on the experiment and how it turned out (e.g., you may find yourself criticizing how well you conducted the experiment rather than considering the outcome of testing out Hypothesis B).

It might be helpful to take a quick look back over Module 19 if you need some refreshing around the compassionate self-practice, and take a few minutes to use this practice to step into this compassionate mindset before engaging in each of the steps just mentioned.

Self-Reflective Questions

How easy or difficult was it to design your experiment? Why do you think this was?

_____

_____

_____

_____

_____

_____

_____

_____

_____

_____

_____

_____

_____

How was it carrying out the experiment? What difficulties (if any) did you notice? How did you feel emotionally and in your body?

_____

_____

_____

_____

_____

_____

_____

_____

_____

_____

_____

_____

What was the impact on your beliefs at the gut level and at the rational level? How do you understand this? What lessons can you draw from your experience that might be helpful for your work with clients?

_____

_____

_____

_____

_____

_____

_____

_____

_____

_____

_____

_____

_____

_____

How did you find using your compassionate self to guide the process of the experiment? Did you have any difficulties? If so, what would help with this in the future?

_____

_____

_____

_____

_____

_____

_____

_____

_____

_____

_____

_____

_____

_____

PART III

Developing the Flows of Compassion

MODULE 23

Compassion from Self to Others: Skill Building Using Memory

The next few modules focus on different "flows" of compassion. As we've discussed, the idea of flow relates to the different directions in which compassion can be focused, expressed, and experienced. This module addresses compassion flowing outward from self to others; it is an opportunity to practice focusing on and acting from the mindset of your compassionate self when directing compassion to others. Compassion for others is often regarded as an inherent and natural part of the therapist's role, and is often the "easier" flow of compassion with which therapists identify and connect. However, compassion for others can prove more complicated than is sometimes appreciated. The next few modules feature practices to help you connect with this flow and become more familiar with how it operates within you.

Compassion Flowing Out from Memory

This practice involves focusing on a memory of acting compassionately toward another person. Memories are a good place to begin cultivating compassion, because they can help us connect with and build upon our lived experiences of compassion and the feelings that go with these experiences. Working with memory is a way of engaging with mental imagery to stimulate our minds and bodies in intentional ways. The more we practice such imagery exercises, the easier it is to utilize the systems in our brain that facilitate compassion and that will help us work with our threat systems (Gilbert, 2010).

This first exercise gets us in touch with the experience of bringing compassion to another person; to become more aware of the presence and influence of compassionate motivation as it shapes our minds and influences our felt emotions and bodily sensations.

The exercise allows us to experience how the compassionate self operates in us as we direct care toward other people.

In the following practice, you can use a memory of being compassionate toward a client with whom you've worked, or a memory involving a friend, family member, or other person. The key is to select a memory of a situation in which you acted out of genuine compassion to help activate compassionate feelings within you. As with the previous exercises, realize that it may take time for your feelings of compassion to develop; continue to focus on your compassionate intention and wishes for the other person even if the compassionate feelings themselves may take time to arise.

 EXERCISE. Compassion Flowing Out from Memory

1. Find a quiet place where you are unlikely to be disturbed and engage in a few moments of soothing rhythm breathing. Adopt the relaxed, dignified posture and friendly facial expression that you associate with your compassionate self.

2. Bring to mind a memory of a time when you were caring and compassionate toward another person who was struggling or suffering, perhaps one of your clients. Try not to choose a memory in which the other person experienced extreme distress. Elaborate on the memory by picturing the scene in your mind. Imagine your surroundings and how the other person looked and sounded.

3. Imagine yourself at your compassionate best, demonstrating and embodying qualities of strength, wisdom, kindness, and commitment. Imagine how you might appear when embodying these qualities as your compassionate self. Adapt your posture to help you express these qualities.

4. Focus on the sensations and emotions in your body as you remember feeling kindness and care toward this person. Connect these feelings with your friendly facial expression.

5. Focus on your intention to be caring and supportive of this person. Allow yourself to be sensitive to his or her experience of suffering, and meet the suffering with a sense of confidence in your ability to be helpful. Experience a desire for the person to be free of suffering and to flourish. Allow any feelings of warmth to expand in your body.

6. Focus on your compassionate tone of voice and the wise and kind things you said or wanted to say to this person. Think of the compassionate things you did or wanted to do, and notice how this makes you feel.

7. Spend time focusing on your pleasure in being able to express compassion and be kind and helpful.

8. When you are ready, allow the image to fade and return your attention to your soothing rhythm breathing. Open your eyes and readjust back to your environment.

After finishing the exercise, take a moment to reflect on your experience of the practice and the feelings it brought up for you, as demonstrated in Erica's example.

EXAMPLE: Erica's Reflection of Compassion Flowing Out from Memory

> **What was your experience? What occurred in your mind and body during the exercise? What emotions did you experience? How did it leave you feeling? Did your experiences change during the exercise?**
>
> *At first, I struggled to find a memory I could focus on. I immediately thought of clients I've had difficulty with, but I understand this as my threat system doing its work. I settled on a therapy session I'd had with Sarah. It was the first time she had spoken about the loss of her father, and I created space for her to connect with her sadness. She was in floods of tears, and I could see how brave she was being in sharing her grief with me. I kept encouraging her to stay with her experiences. I felt strong and stable for her, and imagined myself looking upright and attentive. I imagined the warmth I felt for her flowing out with my breath. I softened and slowed my voice, conveying a sense of acceptance and care. I can remember noticing impulses to step in and fix things, but I let these urges pass, knowing what she needed most. It felt good to remember being helpful and to focus on her benefiting from our work. I was left with a feeling of warmth in my chest.*

Now, take a moment to consider your own experience of the exercise and the feelings it brought up in you:

 EXERCISE. My Compassion Flowing Out from Memory

> **What was your experience? What occurred in your mind and body during the exercise? What emotions did you experience? How did it leave you feeling? Did your experiences change during the exercise?**

Self-Reflective Questions

Reflecting on what occurred for you during this exercise, to what extent did you experience the different attributes of the first psychology of compassion (sensitivity, sympathy, distress tolerance, empathy, nonjudgment, care for well-being)? Did you experience some of these attributes more strongly than others?

_____

_____

_____

_____

_____

_____

_____

_____

_____

_____

_____

_____

_____

_____

Did any obstacles come up during the exercise? If so, how did you work with them?

_____

_____

_____

_____

_____

_____

_____

_____

_____

_____

_____

_____

_____

_____

How might your experience in this module be relevant for clients who are having difficulty experiencing compassion for others? What might you do with them?

_____

_____

_____

_____

_____

_____

_____

_____

_____

_____

_____

_____

_____

Compassion from Self to Others: Skill Building Using Imagery

In the previous module, you connected with a memory of providing compassion to another person, and noticed the feelings that came up while doing so. This module focuses on developing the self-to-other flow of compassion through focusing compassion on the people around us, including people we are indifferent to and those we find difficult. This exercise is an adapted version of the loving-kindness meditations practiced in Buddhist traditions (e.g., Salzberg, 2002). The practice is also known as *Metta Bhavana*, which can be translated as cultivation or development (*Bhavana*) of kindness, friendliness, and nonromantic love (*Metta*). In this meditation we bring a kind, compassionate attitude to other people in four stages:

1. To people we know and love.
2. To people we know less well.
3. To people we find difficult.
4. And, ultimately, to all sentient beings.

The practice involves focusing on the basic connection we have with other people and our shared human aspirations and experiences. Because the practice is based around developing unconditional compassion for others, it also allows us to notice and work with our natural tendencies to judge, criticize, and reject particular people, or even relate critically to our own feelings toward them. In this sense, it can help us become aware of the activation of the threat system when relating to other people, while also providing practice in shifting the focus of our attention to one of stimulating compassion for ourselves and others in mutually beneficial ways.

The practice provides a means to cultivate various facets of compassion for others, reminiscent of the two psychologies of compassion presented earlier. These include *engagement* with the reality of suffering in others coupled with the genuine desire and *aspiration* that they be free of such suffering. Importantly, it also involves the hope and wish that others actively flourish, experiencing happiness and prosperity.

When we encounter difficulty or resistance as we bring compassion to others, it can be helpful to adopt a mindful awareness of how these reactions play out in our bodies and minds. We don't have to pretend to be compassionate, but we *can* choose to bring a kindly curious, wise interest to any resistance that arises within us, while reaffirming our aspiration for the well-being of others, or perhaps aspiring that we, in the future, can connect to such wishes and sentiments for other people (e.g., "Even though I cannot open to this person at present, I can aspire to be more open to caring for this person in the future").

 EXERCISE. Focusing Compassion onto Others

Adopt a posture that is comfortable yet alert and begin your soothing rhythm breathing. Create a friendly facial expression and allow your eyes to close if this feels comfortable.

Now imagine that you are identifying with your compassionate self. Bring to mind the qualities of your compassionate self: warmth, wisdom, strength, and commitment. Imagine these qualities vividly within you. Practice hearing your voice, in your own mind, as kind and encouraging.

SOMEONE YOU ARE CLOSE TO

Bring to mind someone you care about and feel close to: a person you naturally feel warmly toward. Imagine this person before you—how he or she looks, sounds, and moves about in the world. You might imagine the person in a visual image, or just create a felt sense of him or her being present with you.

Now imagine a time when this person went through a difficult event or experience. Allow yourself to be sensitive to his or her suffering and to empathize with his or her experiences. Notice your feelings of care and concern for this person, allowing compassion to arise naturally. Notice your motivation to be helpful and to alleviate this person's suffering.

From the perspective of your compassionate self (maintaining your friendly facial expression and warm tone of voice), imagine sending the following heartfelt wishes to this person:

- *May you be happy and well,* [say this person's name].
- *May you be free of suffering and pain,* [say this person's name].
- *May you experience joy and well-being,* [say this person's name].

Repeat the above sequence for the following minute, connecting to the flow of compassion toward this person. Bring your attention to how you feel when expressing these wishes. Imagine them experiencing the positive states you are wishing for them, and notice the feelings that come up in you as you imagine this. If you have any difficulties in the flow of your feelings toward him or her, kindly notice these and reconnect with your intention and motivation to be compassionate, kind, and committed.

Allow the image to fade and focus on your soothing rhythm breathing.

SOMEONE WHO IS NEUTRAL

Now think of a client or someone else for whom you feel neutrally, someone you neither like nor dislike. It might be a person you have only met briefly, or someone with whom you have limited but regular contact (e.g., a shop assistant, work colleague).

As you bring this person to mind, reflect on the compassionate insight that, just like you, this person finds him- or herself in the flow of life, with difficult emotions and a mind that is hard to manage. Just like you and the people close to you, this person has hopes, dreams, and is trying to be happy and to be loved, despite life's setbacks and disappointments. This person, like you, has been shaped by many circumstances outside of his or her control.

Now imagine this person experiencing suffering, such as feeling lonely or disappointed. Allow yourself to feel concern and care, connecting to his or her suffering and empathizing with his or her difficult experiences. For the next minute, repeat the following wishes and hopes for the person:

- *May you be happy and well,* [say this person's name].
- *May you be free of suffering and pain,* [say this person's name].
- *May you experience joy and well-being,* [say this person's name].

Bring awareness to how you feel when articulating these wishes. There might be a natural flow of concern and care, or you might find yourself feeling indifferent, uncertain, anxious, or frustrated. Notice how your reactions feel in your body. Try to bring a curious and mindful awareness to all of the experiences that arise in you, perhaps observing, with kind interest, the ways in which your compassionate motivation and your threat system are conflicting. Gently return to your compassionate aspirations for this person. Imagine them experiencing the positive states you are wishing for them, and notice the feelings that come up in you as you imagine this.

Allow the image to fade and focus on your soothing rhythm breathing.

SOMEONE YOU FIND DIFFICULT

Now think of someone you dislike, have had conflict with, or someone with whom you would generally choose not to spend time.

Picture this person in your mind, focusing on the felt sense of his or her presence. As you begin to focus compassion on this person, remember that, like you, he or she is a human being who wants to be happy and to avoid suffering. This person, too, finds him- or herself in the flow of life, with a complex brain shaped by millions of years of evolution and with a sense of self shaped by circumstances outside of his or her control. Like you, this person is doing the best he or she can in the face of life's difficulties. Just like you, this person sometimes suffers with anxiety, anger, and sadness. If memories of things this person has done intrude upon your compassionate reflection, see if it's possible to consider that even these difficult behaviors had a valid basis from the person's point of view—that somehow, from his or her perspective, the behaviors made sense. Allow yourself to also have compassion for yourself, recognizing that it makes sense that you might struggle to feel compassion for this person who may push your own buttons for reasons that aren't your fault.

Now imagine this person experiencing suffering or struggle. See if it's possible to allow yourself to feel moved and connected to his or her suffering and pain, perhaps sensing his or her fear, loneliness, disappointment, or feelings of rejection or failure. Remind yourself that even if the things this person has done are hurtful, he or she has done so in response to pain, to avoid suffering, to pursue happiness, or because he or she had the misfortune of growing up in a situation that taught them to meet their needs in harmful ways. Allow yourself to care for this person as a human being and perhaps to wish that he or she experience the things that will help him or her grow in helpful directions. Keeping your friendly facial expression and your warm voice tone, imagine directing the following heartfelt wishes toward this person:

- *May you be happy and well,* [say this person's name.]
- *May you be free of suffering and pain,* [say this person's name.]
- *May you experience joy and well-being,* [say this person's name.]

As you repeat the statements, visualize this person in your mind. Focus on your desire for this person to be happy and to flourish, connecting to the phrases as you direct them toward him or her. Imagine them experiencing the positive states you are wishing for them, and notice the feelings that come up in you as you imagine this. Notice how the exercise makes you feel. You might notice an easy flow of care and concern, or you might become aware of resentment, anger, or an absence of feeling. Notice how these experiences resonate in your body. There is no right or wrong way to feel. Bring an open, kind, and mindful curiosity to what you are experiencing, perhaps noticing your own threat system becoming active to protect you, and recognizing how it makes sense that this might happen.

Reaffirm your intention to open your heart and mind to this person and commit to your intention that he or she experience compassion. Focus on the humanity of the person, on his or her similarities with other humans and with you. You might choose to imagine the person free of the pain or hurt that causes him or her to act in ways that are hurtful to him- or herself and others, including you.

Allow the image to fade, and focus on your soothing rhythm breathing.

ALL LIVING BEINGS

The final part of the exercise asks you to extend compassion to all people. In the stages above, you connected to the basic humanity common to all people: the same yearning to be free of suffering, the same hopes to be happy; the similar fears, pain, emotions, joys, and desires that come with being human; the same experiences that connect people from all walks of life.

Start by contemplating the people you care about, such as your friends and family, one by one, before moving on to people you have less connection with, such as people you walk past on your way to work. Widen your awareness further to include people with whom you experience conflict or difficulty. Remind yourself that all people, just like you, want to be happy and avoid suffering. Just like you, all humans want to be loved and to avoid rejection. Just like you, they want to be safe. Allow your awareness to expand to take in people from your neighborhood and city, people who live in your country, and finally to all living beings everywhere. Imagining all humans, express the following wishes and aspirations:

- *May all living beings be happy and well.*
- *May all living beings be free of suffering and pain.*
- *May all living beings experience joy and well-being.*

Imagine your wishes spreading out to all humanity, as if your compassion could grow and touch each person, inspiring compassion in them in turn, which then spreads to others. Allow yourself to appreciate the interconnectedness of all living beings. Imagine all of these beings receiving your compassionate wishes and being filled with feelings of happiness, freedom from suffering, and well-being.

Let the visualization fade and bring an awareness to how your body feels, noticing the contact points between your body and what supports you. When you are ready, open your eyes and readjust to your environment.

After you have practiced the meditation, write down your experience on page 236. In Erica's example, she has focused specifically on clients, but feel free too focus on people you encounter at work or in your home life, depending on your preference.

EXAMPLE: Erica's Reflection on Focusing Compassion onto Others

What was your experience? What occurred in your mind and body during the exercise? What emotions did you experience? How did the exercise leave you feeling? Did your experiences change during the exercise?

It was a really interesting experience. I found myself thinking about the exercise in terms of the clients I'm seeing.

The first stage was easy. I thought of Paul, who has made such progress with his agoraphobia. I feel our relationship has been an important factor in helping him to make changes. When I thought of him, I could connect with his struggles and my wishes for him to be happy and free of suffering. I was able to take pleasure in thoughts of him doing well, and I noticed a warmth in my chest.

I found the second stage more difficult, as I felt uncomfortable acknowledging that I feel differently toward other clients. I chose Sue, a client I've just started seeing. She has depression, and if I'm honest, I find her hopelessness and lack of motivation frustrating. Starting the exercise with her, I realized how much my heart sinks when I see her appointment in my calendar. I felt guilty thinking this, but was able to refocus on the exercise—and this helped. Spending time focusing on her, and how difficult it must be for her to muster the energy to come to session, I felt moved. Given my experience after my mother died, her lack of energy and motivation made sense to me. It seemed so tragic, all that she has been through, and I found myself feeling sad and heavy in my body. Connecting to the wishes felt affirming. I felt a desire for things to be different for her, and to help her find ways to feel better.

The third person I chose was Sonia, a client I ended up referring to someone else. We just simply didn't click, and she seemed combative and frustrated by my style; she seemed to want someone to tell her what to do, and that's not how I do therapy. I feel so embarrassed just thinking of her. During the exercise I noticed my mind wandering— wanting to explain and justify myself—but I just noticed this and focused on her as a human being: acting out of pain, afraid of not getting better, and feeling a failure again. The conflict stayed with me; it was weird, like two forces wrestling: one wishing her well and the other feeling frustrated (and then feeling guilty for feeling this way). I noticed my body contracting and tension building in my jaw. Coming back to the phrases was helpful and I was able to connect to the wish that she find peace—that the pain that causes her defensiveness could be eased. I was also able to extend that kindness to myself and my reactions, which was surprising. I could feel my whole body softening.

I loved the last part. It felt like these ripples of feeling expanding and expanding in me.

EXERCISE. My Experience of Focusing Compassion onto Others

What was your experience? What occurred in your mind and body during the exercise? What emotions did you experience? How did the exercise leave you feeling? Did your experiences change during the exercise?

Self-Reflective Questions

Reflecting on your experience of this exercise, are there any implications for the way you prepare for therapy?

_____

_____

_____

_____

_____

_____

_____

_____

_____

How do you think this kind of meditation practice will translate to your work with clients who are having difficulty being compassionate toward others? Thinking about your clients, whom might it suit? Whom might it not suit? What's your reasoning?

_____

_____

_____

_____

_____

_____

_____

_____

_____

Compassion from Self to Others:
Compassionate Behavior

The final exercise in the self-to-other flow of compassion involves practicing and recording compassionate behavior toward other people. As we've discussed, acts of care and compassion can involve engaging in situations that stimulate our threat protection and drive systems. Compassionate acts are not specific to situations and behaviors involving soothing and safeness. In fact, some of the most courageous acts of care involve actively facing danger and threat; think of the firefighter entering a burning building to save a family, or a child standing up to a bully on his or her friend's behalf. What is common in such acts is the compassionate motivation that underpins them.

The three-systems model provides a good framework for considering the impact of our interactions on other people (i.e., which emotion system might be stimulated in them as a result of their interaction with us). This is particularly important when considering how we interact with clients. The ways in which we relate to, think about, and approach other people can also have a powerful impact on our own emotion regulation systems and can prime specific behaviors (e.g., the threat system "prepares" attack–avoidance–appeasing behaviors). If we imagine therapy being carried out by a therapist and client who are both stuck in their threat systems, we might see an interactive dance of defensiveness and avoidance, rather than the provision of a safe base from which to do the difficult work of therapy. In this sense, cultivating compassion for others is of mutual benefit to both self and others, particularly in the way that compassion influences our interactions (e.g., Hutcherson et al., 2008).

The idea of "skillfulness" is also worth considering in the context of compassionate behavior. We might have good intentions, but our actions might be misjudged, inappropriate, or lacking in competency, bringing about unhelpful and unwanted consequences. For example, when approaching a colleague who has just returned from bereavement leave and who is about to start her first session with a client, the most skillful action might *not* be asking her how she is feeling. Our most skillful compassionate actions are grounded in empathy as well as sympathy, and they demonstrate our ability to be sensitive and attuned to what the other person needs at this moment. In this example, what is needed might involve inviting this colleague to meet for coffee at the end of the day to allow her to speak more freely, while also sharing a kind word to show her that she is being held positively in your mind. Using the example of grief, skillful behavior might also require a recognition of our own limits and a willingness not to try to "fix" or "solve" the person's pain, particularly when an effort to do so might increase his or her suffering. This recognition, in turn, might require distress tolerance for our own feelings of inadequacy or anxiety around wanting to be helpful but not knowing how. As we've explored in previous modules, compassionate actions require the key components of *sensitivity* to suffering and *motivation* to relieve it, but they also involve *competencies* and *discernment* about which actions are truly skillful and helpful.

Page 240 features a worksheet for recording your compassionate actions toward other people and your accompanying reflections. There are seven rows on which to record a compassionate action for each day of the week, but you can use the worksheet in whatever way you find helpful (e.g., feel free to record more than one compassionate action per day). Try to create a daily habit of engaging in and reflecting upon your compassionate behaviors, perhaps giving yourself a set time for such reflection.

 EXAMPLE: Erica's Compassionate Behavior Record

Day and date	Description of your compassionate action toward others	Reflection
	Briefly describe your compassionate action (e.g., What did you do? Where did it take place? What was the situation? Who was involved?).	Comment on your experience (e.g., How did you feel? What impact did it have on you and/or others? Would you do it again? Did you learn anything new about yourself or others?).
Monday 3/11/2016	My work colleague told me about a challenging meeting he had just attended. I listened to him without judgment.	I felt happy that my colleague was calmer after our conversation and was able to let go of what was bothering him. Sometimes just listening to someone can make a difference.
Tuesday 3/12/2016	When carrying out exposure work with a client who was afraid of needles, I encouraged her to stay in the room when she wanted to leave. She became angry, but we worked through it together, and she remained in the room for the full session.	It felt difficult at first and I noticed my threat system in action: worrying about upsetting the client, what she might think of me, and what kind of person I was being. But I'm realizing that compassion is not about soothing away distress, but about helping people to face and work with the causes of their suffering. I thought about myself as acting out of care for her—doing what she needed, rather than taking the easy option. I felt stronger thinking of it this way.

EXERCISE. My Compassionate Behavior Record

Day and date	Description of your compassionate action toward others	Reflection
	Briefly describe your compassionate action (e.g., What did you do? Where did it take place? What was the situation? Who was involved?).	Comment on your experience (e.g., How did you feel? What impact did it have on you and/or others? Would you do it again? Did you learn anything new about yourself or others?).

Self-Reflective Questions

How was it to focus specifically on your compassionate behavior toward others during the last week? What did you notice? Did anything surprise you?

_____

_____

_____

_____

_____

_____

_____

_____

_____

_____

Did you experience any personal blocks or difficulties during the last week, or with other elements of the three compassion-for-other modules? How did you understand and work with them?

_____

_____

_____

_____

_____

_____

_____

_____

_____

_____

_____

_____

When you bring to mind your experiences during the compassion-for-other modules, have the exercises given you any new insights into the nature of compassion? Are there any implications for you as a therapist?

_____

_____

_____

_____

_____

_____

_____

_____

_____

_____

_____

Can you think of a specific client for whom working on the compassion-for-others flow might be helpful? Reflecting on your own experience, what might be the best way to introduce these exercises to your clients? How might you help them explore the importance of this flow of compassion?

_____

_____

_____

_____

_____

_____

_____

_____

_____

_____

_____

What have you learned during this module that feels important to remember? This learning might apply for you in your personal life or in your role as a therapist. Are there any learning points that are important for you both personally and professionally?

_____

_____

_____

_____

_____

_____

_____

_____

_____

_____

_____

_____

_____

Compassion from Others to Self: Skill-Building Using Memory

The second flow of compassion involves compassion flowing in from another person to oneself. We've had conversations with numerous therapists who report that, whereas they feel good about their ability to experience compassion *for* others, they struggle to receive and rely upon compassion directed to them *from* others who care about them, even when they may very much need it. Opening ourselves to compassion from others can sometimes activate a number of fears and blocks in us, for understandable reasons. The next couple of modules focus on cultivating our receptivity to compassion in much the same way any new skill is cultivated: with training, practice, and patience. Such exploration can also help us better understand the struggles our clients can have in believing and accepting the compassion we direct to them in therapy.

Compassion Flowing In from Memory

The first practice involves focusing on a memory of receiving kindness or care from other people. As you experienced in Module 23, you'll use your memory to stimulate experiences of soothing, safeness, and affiliation with others. The exercise also allows us to focus on being positively held in another person's mind, preparing us to be open and attentive to these experiences in the future. Finally, the exercise provides an opportunity for you to notice your experience of what it's like to focus on receiving compassion from others, and to reflect upon any blocks or resistance that might arise in doing this.

When choosing a memory to work with, try not to pick a time when you felt a complex mix of emotions or experienced significant distress (otherwise your mind, courtesy of your tricky threat-focused brain, may be drawn to focus on the distress rather than the experience of compassion). You might start by picking an occasion in which someone went out of his or her way to help you (e.g., when a friend offered to help you move), before moving on to more emotionally powerful memories. As you progress through the exercise, focus on the mind of the other person and his or her desire and motivation to be helpful and kind to you. Focus also on how you experience what is being offered to you in your own mind and body, allowing a sense of warmth, gratitude, and pleasure to arise. As with previous exercises, if you find such feelings absent or difficult to access, you might experiment with focusing on how it would feel *if you did* have such experiences.

 EXERCISE. Compassion Flowing In from Memory

1. Start with some soothing rhythm breathing, adopting an upright, comfortable, and alert posture. Close your eyes, and create a friendly facial expression as if meeting someone you cared about.

2. When you are ready, bring to mind a memory of a time when someone behaved in a kind or caring manner toward you. Re-create the event in your mind by focusing on your various senses: What did you see, hear, smell, or feel?

3. Now focus on the person's desire and motivation to be helpful, supportive, and kind to you. How did this kindness or care show itself? Spend time focusing on the following:
   - The kind or caring facial expressions of the person in your memory.
   - The things the person said and the tone of his or her voice.
   - The feelings in the other person: what he or she felt for you and wanted for you at that moment.
   - The way the person acted or related to you: what he or she did to be helpful or kind.

4. As you recall the memory, allow yourself to feel gratitude and pleasure in receiving this kindness. If this is difficult for you to do, just try to imagine what it would feel like *if you were able* to experience such gratitude and joy. Imagine the person's compassion registering with you and imagine how it would feel to be held positively in his or her mind. Experiment with your own body posture and facial expression to give you a sense of the kindness and care that you are recalling.

5. In your own time, gently allow the memory to fade and return your focus to your breathing. Open your eyes and readjust to your present environment.

After finishing the exercise, use the space provided in the next exercise to reflect on your experience. Fatima's example captures the way in which our attention, even while focusing on a memory of kindness, can become drawn toward threatening aspects of the experience (in this case, a sense of missing her grandmother and the thought of returning home alone). The example also demonstrates how distractions can be worked with using mindfulness skills we've explored in previous modules.

EXAMPLE: Fatima's Experience of Compassion Flowing In from Memory

---

What was your experience? What did you imagine? What did you notice in your body and emotions?

I immediately thought of my grandmother. A mixture of different memories came up, and I focused on how she greeted me whenever I came by for a visit. A big hug, a cup of tea together . . . I was always touched by how much she remembered about what I was doing and how interested she was. During the exercise, I focused on her smile, the sense of being valued and listened to. And the warmth and smell of the kitchen, the feeling of being safe and cared about.

It did start to make me feel a bit sad that I don't get to see her anymore— she passed away when I was an undergraduate. For a minute or so my mind kept wandering, but I kept bringing my focus back to my grandmother: seeing and feeling her smile, smelling the food, sensing her with me.

 EXERCISE. My Experience of Compassion Flowing In from a Memory

---

What was your experience? What did you imagine? What did you notice in your body and emotions?

Compare and Contrast

One helpful way to explore the impact and potential benefit of compassionate focusing is to contrast the experiences you noted in the preceding exercise with how you might feel if you focused on someone being *unkind* to you. You might want to experiment by briefly bringing to mind a recent argument or disagreement and noticing how this memory influences how you feel. It might be interesting to consider how often, on an average day, we imagine, recall, or anticipate people treating us unkindly, remembering that our evolved brains, biased as they are toward detecting and responding to potential threats, are more likely to focus our attention on such experiences than on positive ones. Luckily, we can choose to purposefully bring to mind memories that can help prompt the sorts of emotional states that we'd like to have.

Working with Blocks

As in Fatima's example, you may have discovered that the exercise highlighted particular blocks or fears in relation to receiving compassion from others. As we see with Fatima, such blocks could include a sense of loneliness, grief, or sadness that you don't have the kind of relationships you would like in your current life. Or the exercise might have triggered memories of relationships or interactions in which the quality of kindness was lacking. Just imagining how we are held in another person's mind can create feelings of vulnerability, embarrassment, and shame that can activate the threat system and reduce our receptivity to compassion, particularly if we experience attachment anxiety. It is common to have reactions to compassion that derive from implicitly held associations stemming from our past experience with attachment figures (Gilbert 2010). In this way, opening to compassion or connectedness involves opening to our attachment history—which can, understandably, be painful for many people (e.g., see Bowlby, 1980).

The important point to note is that nothing is going wrong. These experiences are not a sign that compassion isn't for you or that an exercise isn't working—in fact, it can mean quite the opposite. Learning to work with blocks, fears, and resistances to compassion is in many ways the focus of CFT as a psychotherapy, and these experiences can point us toward areas in which we can grow. These obstacles to receiving care from others (and in turn, giving care to ourselves) can be the very things blocking our clients' access to their safeness and soothing system (and our own). Understanding why such blocks and fears have arisen and working skillfully with them as they arise (e.g., by connecting with the mindset of your compassionate self, and imagining how this version of you would relate to these experiences) are integral parts of the therapeutic process.

Self-Reflective Questions

Did you experience any blocks or resistances during the exercise? What did you notice? How did you experience them?

_____

_____

_____

_____

_____

_____

_____

_____

_____

_____

_____

_____

If you did notice any blocks, how did you work with them?

_____

_____

_____

_____

_____

_____

_____

_____

_____

_____

_____

_____

_____

_____

Whether or not you experienced any blocks to receiving compassion from others, what can you take from this exercise that might be helpful in your work with clients?

_____

_____

_____

_____

_____

_____

_____

_____

_____

_____

_____

_____

_____

_____

MODULE 27

Compassion from Others to Self: Opening to Kindness from Others

The second exercise targeting the other-to-self flow of compassion is a daily practice that involves opening to kindness and compassion from others. In many ways, this is a practice of attention—bringing attention to these acts of kindness from others and the experiences they evoke in us. As discussed previously, our brains have a natural negativity bias that helped ensure our ancestors' survival: These brains place a high priority on scanning for, registering, and recalling threat and danger. The aim of the current exercise is not to supress or ignore negative interpersonal experiences, but to help our brains balance this bias. We can intentionally choose to "take in" the good that occurs to us, savoring it in our awareness, until the event becomes a full, rich experience for us (Hanson & Mendius, 2009).

Such savoring might involve acknowledging and dwelling on the intention of the person who has been compassionate toward us, opening to the sense of being held positively in his or her mind. It might involve exploring the various qualities of feeling and emotion the interaction has created in you, allowing sensations to build and unfold in your body (e.g., a spreading sense of warmth in the chest). With practice, such focusing can become a habit of mind; we can learn to pay attention to these events, however small, as they occur in our daily lives. Rather than engaging in a formal practice as you've done with many of the other exercises, this will involve you spending a week (or more, if you like) trying to notice and record experiences of receiving kindness from others. Keeping track of such experiences can help us train our minds to notice them in the future. In doing this, it can be helpful to connect with the perspective of your compassionate self. Let's take a look at Erica's example of her daily practice.

EXAMPLE: Erica's Opening to Kindness from Others Worksheet

Day of the week	What I noticed about the other person's kind behavior toward me (*external*)	What I experienced, and focused on, in my emotions, body, and mind (*internal*)
Monday	A client bought me a card at her final session. Her words were really touching, and she thanked me for my support and encouragement.	I really tried to connect with her words. I can be quick to skip over "thank-yous," but I let myself really listen. I read over the words a few times during the day. It made me cry, but I was OK with that.
Tuesday	A stranger smiled and held the door open for me at the leisure center.	Warmth in my body, a sense of gratitude.
Wednesday	My supervisor phoned, checking how I was doing with a difficult client. She made time for me and was patient and kind.	I felt cared about—that someone else had been thinking of me during the week. She's really busy, so I felt touched that she gave me her time. I allowed myself to breathe.
Thursday	My friend Suzanne left me a voicemail inviting me out this weekend. She said she was looking forward to seeing me again. Her voice was warm and genuine.	I was planning to spend the weekend in, and initially felt frustrated by the call. But I was able to be mindful of these thoughts, and I refocused on Suzanne's voice and words. I let myself feel thankful and appreciative for her contact, and remembered my intention to reengage with my social life. I smiled when I imagined seeing her face. I felt my body soften.
Friday	One of my colleagues, Paul, brought me a mocha—my favorite coffee drink—without my asking. He gently put his hand on my shoulder as he put it on my desk.	I really needed it! I stopped my work and let myself enjoy the drink. I focused on the warmth of the cup in my hand and the warmth I felt toward Paul.
Saturday	I met Suzanne in town and she paid for lunch as a treat. She asked about my Mom and how I am doing without pushing me. She looked concerned and interested.	I let myself be treated! It felt good! Suzanne really knows me, and it was helpful to talk. I worried about being overwhelmed, but I felt safe sharing with her. I noticed feeling lighter in my chest. I felt cared for.
Sunday	One of the neighbors crossed the road to say hello when I was out shopping. She seemed really pleased to see me, and asked me to stop by for coffee during the week.	When I saw her, I felt anxious as I hadn't seen anyone all day and was in my own world. But her friendliness was infectious. I felt better for smiling and talking. I focused on feeling part of the local community and connected to people in the area.

Use the worksheet on the following pages to record your daily practice of noticing the kindness that others give you, and the experiences that arise in you as a result.

✍ EXERCISE. My Opening to Kindness from Others Worksheet

Day of the week	What I noticed about the other person's kind behavior toward me (*external*)	What I experienced, and focused on, in my emotions, body, and mind (*internal*)
Monday		
Tuesday		
Wednesday		

Thursday		
Friday		
Saturday		
Sunday		

Self-Reflective Questions

How did experiencing compassion from other people affect you? That is, what were your emotional or physical reactions, and did they change or grow during the course of your practice?

_____

_____

_____

_____

_____

_____

_____

_____

_____

_____

_____

What was it like to write down the experiences (if you did)? Were you able to do this? Did you forget? Did any blocks, fears, or difficult reactions get in the way? Was there any uneasiness? What stood out for you?

_____

_____

_____

_____

_____

_____

_____

_____

_____

_____

_____

_____

If there were blocks, fears, or difficult reactions, how did you work with them? How might you compassionately work with them in the future?

_____

_____

_____

_____

_____

_____

_____

_____

_____

_____

_____

_____

Have the exercises given you any insight into your own relationships and how you experience compassion and care from other people? What do these insights mean to you? What might you try differently in the future?

_____

_____

_____

_____

_____

_____

_____

_____

_____

_____

_____

_____

In the light of your experience of the compassion-flowing-in exercises, how might you integrate them into your clinical practice? Do you have clients for whom such practices might be helpful? How might you introduce them to these clients? What rationale might you give?

_____

_____

_____

_____

_____

_____

_____

_____

_____

_____

_____

_____

MODULE 28

Compassion Flowing to the Self: Compassionate Letter Writing

In the previous few modules, you've explored directing compassion to others and receiving compassion directed from others to yourself. The third flow of compassion in CFT is self-compassion: the ability to experience and direct compassion toward ourselves, as well as to receive and benefit from it. Hopefully this will feel somewhat familiar to you, as we attempted to set the stage for self-compassion in the early modules, with more formal introduction to some self-compassion practices presented in Module 7 (considering how your struggles make sense in light of your developmental history), and Module 20 (directing compassion from the perspective of your compassionate self to a struggling version of the self). In this module, we explore self-compassion from another angle: that of compassionate letter writing. The idea is to help ourselves develop a repertoire of methods for being able to engage warmly and compassionately with ourselves (and to help our clients do the same) when faced with challenging problems.

Crafting a Compassionate Letter

There are many ways to orient a compassionate letter. Perhaps one of the most common is to write a letter from the perspective of your compassionate self to a version of the self that is struggling or suffering—perhaps around an issue you've observed yourself struggling with either in the past or in an ongoing way in your current life. You'll begin by revisiting the compassionate-self practice to help you reconnect with this caring, wise, and courageous perspective, and then you'll write a compassionate letter designed to support and encourage you in working with a personal problem or challenge. It might be useful for you now to remind yourself of the familiar struggle you identified earlier (or, if you prefer, one that has arisen in your life more recently).

Using that challenging problem as an anchor point, let's take a moment to refamiliarize ourselves with the two psychologies of compassion—*engagement with suffering* and *preparing and acting to alleviate and prevent it*—that you'll draw upon in writing the letter. First, let's revisit the six qualities of compassionate engagement, as well as some possible language through which these qualities might be expressed in such a letter:

- *Care for well-being:* "I want you to know that I care about you."
- *Sensitivity:* "If you're reading this, you're probably suffering or having a hard time right now."
- *Sympathy:* "It's hard to know that you're hurting, and I want you to know that you're not alone."
- *Empathy:* "From experience, I know you're likely feeling a lot of different emotions, such as frustration, anxiety, and shame. Give yourself permission to notice what you're feeling."
- *Non-judgment:* "I want to remind you that it isn't your fault that you're having a hard time right now, and that these struggles are part of having a human life."
- *Distress tolerance:* "And although it's hard, I also want to remind you that there are things you might try which could make this situation a bit easier to bear."

One of the useful things about having our clients write a compassionate letter to themselves (and doing so ourselves) is that each of us is the expert on what we most need when we're struggling, and what would be most helpful. So, when crafting a compassionate letter, the idea is to draw upon this wisdom to communicate understanding, validation, support, encouragement, and suggestions that, based on our experience, are most likely to be helpful to us. It's also important that the "tone of voice" in the letter be infused with warmth.

In proceeding with the letter, you can then move on to the second psychology of compassion: reminding yourself of things that might be helpful to this struggling version of yourself as you work with this difficulty, as well as concrete suggestions about things that, from your experience, are likely to be helpful in preparing you to address this challenge. Here are some examples of such elements that might be included a compassionate letter:

- Reminders of things that you find soothing or helpful.
- Reminders to connect with people to whom you are close or whom you know will support you.
- Reminders that might help this struggling version of you to shift into a compassionate mindset.
- Practical suggestions of things you've found helpful in the past (e.g., breaking things down into small steps, specific coping behaviors that have worked for you).

- Suggestions around self-care behaviors (e.g., exercise, breathing).
- Encouragement and reminders of previous successful coping efforts ("I know that you can do this; you've faced difficult situations before and have managed them well"), and of why you're making efforts to improve—anchoring this effort to values that are important to you.
- Suggestions that might broaden your awareness of your feelings and help you become tolerant and understanding of them.

As an example, let's look at Fatima's letter:

Dear Fatima,

If you're reading this, you're probably feeling pretty terrible right now. Maybe something has happened with Alex or another client that has triggered feelings of inadequacy in you, or you're struggling with something else. I want you to know that I care about you, and that I'm not the only one. Given your history of being criticized, it makes sense that it would be really upsetting when you encounter disapproval or things don't go as you hoped, doesn't it? You were criticized a lot growing up, which taught you to blame yourself first, even for things that weren't your fault.

But here's the thing: You are a committed, dedicated therapist, and even the fact that you are upset about this is a testament to how much you care about your clients and want to do a good job helping them. See if it's possible to take the kindness, compassion, and understanding you show your clients every day, and give some of it to yourself. Even if right now you feel like you don't deserve it, you know that doing this will help you feel better so that you can be there for them as well.

*See if it's possible to look kindly at the feelings you're having, and try to understand how they make sense, remembering that everyone struggles with difficult feelings sometimes. **There is nothing wrong with you.** Try to make room for those feelings, accept them, and then consider what might be helpful in working with them and in coping with the problem that triggered them.*

Remember that there are lots of things you can do that have been helpful in the past. Try doing some soothing rhythm breathing, safe-place imagery, listen to some hip-hop, or watch an episode of "Friends"—that always helps you feel comfortable and brightens your spirits. You can call Rachel or Ariel, or even Erica—you know they will listen to you, understand, and help you feel better. You might also think about going for a run, or treating yourself by getting some Thai food or making some gulab jamun. See if you can get that soothing system working to help balance out the feelings of threat you're having.

Most of all, know that you won't always feel this way. You've been doing a lot of work to improve yourself as a therapist and to learn to have compassion for yourself, and it's working. Some difficult moments in life just need to be survived. You can do it, and I'm here for you!

Love,
Fatima

EXERCISE. Compassionate Letter Writing

Begin by creating a comfortable, quiet setting in which you can be undisturbed for a little while. To write the letter, you might use a favorite pen, if you have one, and select something to write on that you'll have easy access to in the future—perhaps a piece of paper you can fold and put in your day planner, or a cherished journal that you can easily access. Center yourself with soothing rhythm breathing. Allow yourself to shift into the caring, wise, confident perspective of your compassionate self (revisiting the practice in Module 19, if it would be helpful), select the challenging situation you'll be working with, and bring to mind an image of yourself struggling with this situation and the emotions that it brings up in you. Then, reflecting on the previous suggestions and example, write a compassionate letter to yourself, including everything you think might be helpful to you when you next find yourself struggling. Make it as individualized as possible, taking advantage of the things you know about yourself, what you tend to find helpful in such situations, and what would be most helpful for you to hear in such moments of struggle. As when introducing this exercise to our clients, remember that it's important to understand that there's no pressure to "get it right." They can write as many of these letters as they like, and so can you.

Once the letter has been completed, it is useful to reflect on the process. In doing this, we've divided the reflective questions into two sections: one to be completed immediately after the letter is completed, and one to be completed after rereading the letter a few days later. When reading the letter (either aloud or in your imagination), make sure to do so with a compassionate tone of voice that reflects the warmth of its content. Let's take a look at Fatima's example.

 EXAMPLE: Fatima's Reflection: Part I—Immediately upon Writing the Letter

---

What was your experience of writing the letter? What feelings came up for you? What did you notice in your body? What else were you aware of?

Writing the letter was really powerful for me. Initially, it felt a little weird, and I had some reluctance. Each time the exercises have had me visualize a struggling version of myself, it's felt a little strange, but it's getting easier. With patience I was able to do it, and I found that when I was able to imagine myself during those times I've felt really terrible about my work with Alex, I actually did have compassion for that version of myself—I could see how distressed I was about it, and how that distress was related to my strong desire to help her, and to fears that I was failing to do so. That realization helped me feel warmth toward myself, and then the letter just flowed. Once that happened, a feeling of contentment and resolve came up in me—along with a calm, warm feeling in my body. It felt good to shift into a compassionate perspective and think about how I could help myself. I was also surprised that when I started trying to think of what might be helpful for me when I'm in that space, a lot of things came up—when I think about it, there are a lot of things that I find soothing and helpful. It also felt good to remind myself that I do have people in my life who really value me, are understanding, and are there when I need them.

Did any obstacles come up as you wrote the letter? If so, how did you work with them?

As I wrote, initially it felt a little awkward. I found that if I just kept going, I was able to do it, though.

 EXERCISE. Reflecting on Writing the Compassionate Letter, Part I—Immediately upon Writing the Letter

Once you've written your own compassionate letter, complete the following brief reflection.

What was your experience of writing the letter? What feelings came up for you? What did you notice in your body? What else were you aware of?

Did any obstacles come up as you wrote the letter? If so, how did you work with them?

One point we always emphasize to clients is that it's OK to go back and add elements to the letter that might not have occurred to them when writing it, or even to write as many additional letters as they want (e.g., to address different challenges). In the days after writing your letter, feel free to modify it; the only criterion is that the modifications are rooted in a compassionate motivation to make the letter more helpful (rather than, say, self-criticism or perfectionism). After a few days have passed, you'll want to read the letter and reflect on it, as Fatima does next.

 EXAMPLE: Fatima's Reflection, Part II—After Reading the Letter a Few Days Later

> **What was your experience of reading the letter? What feelings and bodily experiences came up for you as your read it?**
>
> *It was surprisingly moving to read the letter. I had a catch in my throat and I got a bit tearful. In writing it, it was clear that I'd drawn on my knowledge of how things play out in me when I struggle, because the letter really spoke to my own soft spots. It was interesting to see how much a letter, especially one written by me to myself, could be so comforting to me, and I could feel my body relaxing as I read it. I should say that I wasn't terribly distressed when I read it (didn't want to wait too long and lose my momentum in working through the modules), but I think it will be very helpful the next time I'm struggling.*
>
>
>
> **Were there any obstacles that came up while reading the letter? If so, how did you work with them?**
>
> *Initially, it felt a bit silly—like "Oh, look, an encouraging letter to me from me!" But I was surprised at how quickly I was drawn into it.*

When you're ready, take a quiet moment to read your compassionate letter to yourself, emphasizing the warm, caring inner voice of your compassionate self. As you read it, see if it's possible to receive the caring you felt when you wrote this letter to yourself—to receive it as a kind message from someone who cares about you and wants to help you. Emphasizing the mental "tone of voice" is important, both because we want the tone of the letter to match that of the compassionate self, and because warm versus harsh voices have very powerful effects upon our emotion regulation systems (Gilbert, 2010).

EXERCISE. My Reflection, Part II—Reading the Compassionate Letter

What was your experience of reading the letter? What feelings and bodily experiences came up for you as your read it?

Were there any obstacles that came up while reading the letter? If so, how did you work with them?

Self-Reflective Questions

What was your overall experience of the letter-writing exercise? What was it like to direct compassion toward, and to receive it from, yourself in this way? What stood out for you?

_____

_____

_____

_____

_____

_____

_____

_____

_____

_____

_____

_____

Has the exercise given you any insight into how you tend to relate to yourself and your ability to direct compassion and care to yourself? What do these insights mean to you? What have you learned that might impact how you do things in the future?

_____

_____

_____

_____

_____

_____

_____

_____

_____

_____

_____

_____

_____

_____

Considering your own experiences, how might you integrate this exercise into your clinical practice? Do you have clients for whom this practice might be helpful? How might you use it with them?

_____

_____

_____

_____

_____

_____

_____

_____

_____

_____

_____

_____

_____

_____

How do your experiences of the self-to-self flow of compassion relate to your understanding of CFT?

_____

_____

_____

_____

_____

_____

_____

_____

_____

_____

_____

_____

_____

_____

PART IV

Engaging Compassionately with Our Multiple Selves

MODULE 29

Getting to Know Our Multiple Selves

In Modules 18 and 19, we explored how different emotions and motives can organize our minds and bodies in very different ways, producing different "versions" of us that pay attention, think, feel, imagine, and are motivated to behave in very different ways. The multiple-selves practice involves getting to know three key emotions as they play through our minds and bodies when considering a recent threatening situation. We refer to these emotions in terms of the "anxious self," the "angry self," and the "sad self" as we explore the ways these different emotions/selves can organize our minds and bodies when they are in the driver's seat. Modern science supports the idea that, rather than having a single "self," our "selves" are made up of multiple, interacting subsystems: different modes of mind shaped by various stages of evolution (Carter, 2008; Teasdale, 1999). This exercise focuses specifically on the mindsets created by emotions we commonly experience when our threat systems are triggered.

The first stage of the exercise involves picking a recent situation in which you experienced a threat-based reaction, and using mental imagery to re-create the scene in your mind's eye. Then pick an emotion (sadness, anxiety, or anger—you might start with the one that stands out most for you) and imagine yourself taking on the emotion as a character or role, as you did previously with the threat-based-self exercise in Module 18 and the compassionate self in Module 19. On this occasion, your role is to personify and embody each emotion as if it were inhabiting your whole being, allowing you to perceive, understand, and consider how you might respond to the situation through the lens of that emotion. It doesn't matter if you did or didn't have awareness of that emotion at the time of the event; the aim of the exercise is to imagine the situation from the mindset of this emotion, *as if* you did experience it. To facilitate this process, try asking yourself this question: "If I fully allowed myself to experience my anxiety/anger/sadness in this situation, how would that affect how I think, feel, and act?" A further question to ask, particularly if you are having difficulty, is "How would I think, feel, and act *if I could* give free reign to my anxiety/anger/sadness in this situation?" The emotional connection can be deepened by taking on the body posture or movements of the corresponding emotional self as you recall the situation in your mind. For example, the "sad self" might have dropped shoulders and a lowered head.

As you move through the exercise, take a few deep breaths between each emotional self, perhaps even bowing or respectfully saying "goodbye" in your mind to each emotion as you allow it to recede, mentally thanking this emotional self for sharing its perspective with you. Don't worry if some emotional selves strive to stick around; if this happens, try to notice them mindfully, compassionately acknowledging that it makes sense that this would happen, before gently continuing to the next "self." Use the grid on page 272 to record your experiences of each emotional self. In the final stage of the exercise, you'll imagine bringing the compassionate self to the situation, and viewing the other selves and the situation from a compassionate perspective. The final square of the grid can then be completed with the experiences of your compassionate self, allowing you to compare and contrast the mindset created by your compassionate motivation to those associated with threat-focused emotions.

Let's take a look at Joe's experience of the multiple-selves exercise:

 EXAMPLE: Joe's Multiple Selves

Joe chose to focus on a recent difficult session of supervision. In the supervision, Joe had brought the case of a client who had questioned the speed of his recovery. When revisiting the scenario in his mind, Joe initially accessed his "angry self," the emotional self that was most prominent at the time. In his mind, he fully embodied his angry self, giving vent to his supervisor. He noticed the feelings of anger returning to his head and shoulders, and even clenched his fists as he recalled the scene. After a few minutes of experiencing his angry self, he opened his eyes and allowed himself a few deeper breaths. Joe stretched, opened his fingers, rolled his shoulders, and wrote down his experiences of his angry self in the grid.

While doubting the presence of other emotions in the scene, he imagined how his "anxious self" might have experienced the supervision if he had paid attention to it and given it voice. Joe was soon able to identify the dread of his supervisor's judgment and the sense of his own stomach knotting. Imagining the scene from his "anxious self's" perspective, Joe connected with a desire to flee the room. He noticed his breathing quicken as he practiced the exercise.

Joe continued the exercise, experiencing the scene from the perspectives of his sad and compassionate selves. Between each "self," he stretched out his body and took a few deep breaths, before making notes in the grid on page 271.

Challenging situation: *Recent supervision when discussing a difficult case.*	
<u>My Angry Self</u>	<u>My Anxious Self</u>
Bodily feelings:	**Bodily feelings:**
Rising tension to my head and shoulders. Agitation. Clenched fists.	*I feel sick in my stomach, lightheaded, and dizzy.* *I'm breathing quickly and lightly.*
Thoughts and images:	**Thoughts and images:**
It is so unfair that I have to have to carry this workload. He knows this, so why is he carrying on like it's all possible? As if he could do any better. I wouldn't want to have him as a therapist—he doesn't listen.	*I'm getting it wrong. I'm going to be humiliated. I'm out of control. Image of myself shaking and being stared at.*
Urges for action:	**Urges for action:**
To criticize my supervisor. To tear into him.	*To avoid talking about the difficulties I'm having and to lie about the client. To leave the room.*
What does this self really want?	**What does this self really want?**
To defend and attack.	*To escape. To hide. To avoid.*
<u>My Sad Self</u>	<u>My Compassionate Self</u>
Bodily feelings:	**Bodily feelings:**
Everything feels heavy. A dropping in my stomach. My head goes down. I feel upset.	*Steady, slowed down. Strong.*
Thoughts and images:	**Thoughts and images:**
I can't get it right. I feel like I'm letting everyone down all the time. I didn't want it to be like this here. My supervisor thinks I'm incompetent, and maybe he's right. Maybe I'm not cut out for this.	*This is a difficult situation and it makes sense that I would feel so strongly. It has been a hard week. There are things I can learn from this supervision and he is actually trying to help.*
Urges for action:	**Urges for action:**
To go home and go to bed.	*To help myself feel safe by slowing my breathing and opening my shoulders. To remind myself of the good intentions that bring me to do this work. To connect back with the supervision.*
What does this self really want?	**What does this self really want?**
To give up. To be on my own.	*To be caring. To work with the difficulty (not shut down).*

Now try the exercise yourself, working through the emotions in turn before accessing your compassionate self. You can choose a personal or clinical example for the exercise, but try and pick a situation in which you felt a degree of strong emotion. The exercise works particularly well with interpersonal situations.

Challenging situation:	
My Angry Self Bodily feelings: Thoughts and images: Urges for action: What does this self really want?	**My Anxious Self** Bodily feelings: Thoughts and images: Urges for action: What does this self really want?
My Sad Self Bodily feelings: Thoughts and images: Urges for action: What does this self really want?	**My Compassionate Self** Bodily feelings: Thoughts and images: Urges for action: What does this self really want?

Emotions about Emotions

When completing the exercise above, you may have noticed that one emotion showed up more strongly for you than others. This happened for Joe: His anger was immediately accessible and dominated his reaction to the situation. You may also have noticed that other emotions were more difficult to access, or that tuning in to a certain emotion was itself very threatening. Growing up, many of our clients may have learned that certain emotions were unacceptable, and may fear or avoid the experience of such feelings. For Joe, acknowledging and exploring the anxiety he experienced in the situation felt both frightening and alien; he hadn't considered the kind of vulnerability he felt during supervision, or the way that part of him wanted to escape and hide. Joe also noticed that thinking about feeling vulnerable in this way shifted him quickly back into anger—at himself ("It's stupid to feel this way.") and at his supervisor ("I can't believe he made me feel like this.").

One way to think about this kind of response is that we can have emotions *about* emotions. We can have anxiety about feeling sad, anger when feeling anxious, anxiety about experiencing anger, and so on (e.g., Greenberg, 2002). Considering such interactions between our emotional "selves" can also give us a window through which to explore emotional dynamics of self-criticism, through considering questions such as "How does your angry self feel about your anxious self?" or "What would your sad self have to say to your angry self?" (Kolts, 2016).

Compassion and the Multiple Selves

Compassion in this sense is not about soothing away distress but about learning to bring awareness to the nature of our suffering and to awaken an intention or desire to do something about it. This might, for example, involve bringing mindful sensitivity to what the "angry self" is *really* up to in our minds: our violent fantasies, rages, impulses to strike out, and the surge of energy to the fists and head. Or it might involve bringing awareness to the anxious self: to the things we are frightened to acknowledge, such as fears of rejection or failure or urges to hide or run away. It might involve acknowledging the sad version of the self, with its desire to shrink, give up, and disappear. With compassion, these aspects of the self that we carry within us can be tolerated, understood, and worked with, rather than being avoided or acted out.

A helpful metaphor when working with multiple selves involves picturing the compassionate self as "captain of the ship" (Kolts, 2011). In the metaphor, the ship is our mind, which has different passengers in the form of the anxious self, the angry self, and the sad self—passengers who haven't been invited aboard, but who serve vital roles in the safe running of the vessel. Although their functions are integral, none of these emotional selves is qualified to captain the ship by itself. The anxious self is a great early-warning alarm system, but only focuses on danger and escape, hiding in times of difficulty and losing track of where the ship intends to go. The angry self is the ship's attack and defense system, but rages and attacks whenever it is feeling vulnerable, or criticizes when things go wrong. The sad self orients the ship toward losses and signals distress, but shrinks and shuts down when overwhelmed. However, the compassionate self—the captain of the ship—is kind, wise, courageous, and competently able to understand all the reactions of the fellow passengers. The compassionate self understands that the passengers are simply trying to do their best, doing the only things they know how to do. With this understanding and sensitivity, the compassionate self is able to reassure the emotional passengers, giving them what they need to feel safe—validation, empathy, support, encouragement—and is able to guide the ship to safety, even when the seas get stormy.

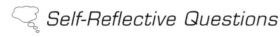 ## *Self-Reflective Questions*

What was your experience of the multiple-selves exercise? Were there any surprises?

_____

_____

_____

_____

_____

_____

_____

_____

_____

_____

_____

_____

_____

Did you notice any strong or difficult reactions to a particular emotional self? Did you notice any avoidance? Did you notice a preference for any particular emotional self? What do those reactions mean to you?

_____

_____

_____

_____

_____

_____

_____

_____

_____

_____

_____

_____

_____

_____

_____

_____

Did your experiences of the multiple-selves exercises have any impact on how you understand yourself? Does this new understanding have any implications for how you understand your own reactions and experiences on a day-to-day basis?

_____

_____

_____

_____

_____

_____

_____

_____

_____

_____

_____

_____

_____

_____

As a therapist, how might the exploration of different emotional selves influence your therapy or supervision? How might you explore this area in the future? Using your experiences of the exercises, how might you work with the impact of your emotional reactions in therapy?

_____

_____

_____

_____

_____

_____

_____

_____

_____

_____

_____

_____

_____

MODULE 30

Writing from the Multiple Selves

This exercise is an extension of the multiple-selves exercise presented in Module 29 but also draws on the extensive literature investigating writing in psychotherapy to aid emotional processing, connection, and expression (e.g., Pennebaker, 1997, 2004). In this exercise, you'll write about a problematic situation from the perspective of each of the emotional selves before using the compassionate self to bring understanding and integration to these emotional perspectives.

EXERCISE. Writing from the Multiple Selves

1. Bring to mind an interpersonal problem. This might be a disagreement or difficulty experienced with a client, work colleague, supervisor, or manager. Avoid selecting a problem with such a high degree of emotion that it would be difficult to deal with during the exercise. In your imagination, provide sensory detail to your experience of the scene: what you saw, heard, smelled, or felt.

2. Next, choose the emotional "self" that was most prominent in your response to the situation (your anxious self, sad self, or angry self). Write about the problem from the perspective of this self, giving full vent to your emotion from that one perspective. Just keep writing for 4–5 minutes, trying not to lift the pen from the page. Don't worry if you repeat yourself or if what you're writing doesn't seem to make sense. Repeated swear words are fine! (This writing exercise is for your eyes only, and should be "stream of consciousness.") The aim is to freely embody and express that emotional self in your writing about the problem. Try and stay true to the emotional self you have chosen: that is, the angry self is *only* ever angry at the subject of its focus. Feel free to focus on both the external aspects of the problematic situation (e.g., how other people are acting) as well any difficult internal experiences present (e.g., the angry self might be angry at *you*—how you felt or what you thought in the situation).

3. Now write about the problem from the perspective of a different emotional self. If you began with anger, write from the experience of your sad or anxious self. Again, write as if expressing a stream of consciousness.

4. Now write about the problem again from the last remaining emotion.

5. Finally, connect with your compassionate self, using the methods you learned earlier in the book. Prepare your body; prepare your mind. Take as long as you need, and when ready, write from the perspective of your compassionate self, drawing upon the various attributes and skills that make up compassion (e.g., caring motivation, sensitivity, sympathy, empathy, distress tolerance, and engaging your wisdom, strength, and commitment). From the perspective of your compassionate self, reflect upon and address the various emotional selves and their reactions before considering how best to work with the situation itself. Consider how the experience and responses of these emotional versions of yourself make sense in the context of your history and the situation (how it is understandable that you would feel anger, anxiety, and/or sadness in relation to this difficult experience). Consider what these emotion-driven versions of you would need to feel safe, and how the compassionate self might support and reassure them. Finally, from the perspective of the compassionate self, reflect on how you might move forward and work with the situation itself.

Now let's consider Erica's example (swear words have been deleted [!], and text edited for length).

 EXAMPLE: Erica's Multiple-Selves Writing Exercise

Situation: A difficult session with Susan (a client with depression) occurring a few weeks ago, on the 6-month anniversary of my mother's death.

Choose the emotion that is most prominent (anxious self/sad self/angry self). From the perspective of the emotional self you have chosen, write about the problem. Write about the external situation as well as your inner experiences (emotions, imagery, thoughts, bodily reactions, motives, etc.).

Chosen self: Anxious self

The session really didn't go well. She was talking and talking and I was just distracted . . . just tense with my thoughts racing all over the place. I think she could tell. I was really struggling that day, and I just didn't want to hear about her mother and her father again. I thought I'd been doing better with this. What if I fall back into how I was feeling right after Mom died? I've got no business doing therapy if I can't even focus on my client.

And this is when I get sad, and I get anxious about getting sad. It feels like it will take over. I can't go there, it's too much. I won't be able to get out of the mood once I'm in it. I'm afraid that I'll get lost in it again. It would ruin my day, my week, and I can't get rid of thoughts about my Mom. I don't want to be thinking about this now . . .

And then I'm back again—what kind of therapist am I if I'm distracting myself like this? What am I going to do?

Now write from another emotional self (anxious/sad/angry).

Chosen self: Angry self

I feel so cross at Susan for going on and on about her family when I'm feeling like this. Why can't she just stop whining and talk about something else? She's lucky to have two parents who are still alive. And having to hear about how hard it is for her to make herself breakfast—I wish I had her problems! She didn't even try to complete her homework; she isn't even trying . . .

I'm angry at myself for even writing this. What kind of terrible therapist thinks these things about her client? I'm supposed to be helping her, and I just want her to shut up.

Now write from another emotional self (anxious/sad/angry).

Chosen self: *Sad self*

My sadness feels so big, I don't know where to start . . .

I feel so alone at the moment. I'm on my own with everything I'm feeling, and everything feels so painful.

I'm sad that I'm not the therapist I used to be. Sometimes it feels like I don't have the energy to keep listening, and I feel like giving up. I do feel sad for Susan and the pain she is feeling. I recognize the hopelessness that she has, but I miss my own family. I miss my relationship. Being with her makes me aware of everything I've lost, things I'll never get back.

Spend as long as you need to access and embody your compassionate self. When you are ready, write from the perspective of your compassionate self, addressing each emotional self as well as the external situation. From this compassionate perspective, how would you understand the perspectives of these emotional selves in relation to this difficult situation? How might you offer understanding, support, and encouragement to each of these emotional selves? How might this kind, wise, courageous, compassionate version of you work with this challenging situation?

It is understandable that I'm anxious, angry, and sad. I've been through a lot in the past year. It has been really hard, and working as a therapist is bound to trigger things for me; it is an unusual job like that. It makes complete sense that I would feel anxious, angry, and sad—even though that is hard to admit even to myself. The truth is that losing loved ones is hard for everyone, and I've been doing much better in recent months. It makes sense that I would struggle on the anniversary of her death, and noticing that I still struggle sometimes doesn't mean I'm a bad therapist—in fact, the fact that I'm concerned about it is a testament to how committed I am to my clients.

I can understand my worries and anxiety as part of my threat system; my mind is just monitoring for danger and the things I fear, trying to protect me. There is nothing going wrong with me. It isn't my fault that my mind goes there, but I can choose how I want to respond.

From my compassionate self, I can see that I still sometimes tend to avoid my sadness and grief. Maybe I'm afraid that my grief will be overwhelming, like it was right after Mom died. That was so scary—I'd never felt like that before, and sometimes it felt like I was trapped in the grief and would never make it out. It makes sense that I'd be afraid of getting stuck there again. Things have gotten much better over time, and I've done a good job lately of reengaging with things I'd pulled back from. It's OK for me to feel a surge of grief sometimes, especially around anniversaries—I wouldn't want to be the sort of person who isn't affected by losing someone I love. The hurt that I'm feeling around this is a sign of my ability to care about and connect with others.

I've been doing better at treating myself as I would treat someone I care about. I just need to keep that up. It's been helpful speaking to my friend Charlotte, who lost her mother last year—maybe it might be helpful to reconnect with her. This is hard for everybody. Mostly, I think it will be helpful to give myself permission to feel whatever I'm feeling, and to keep doing what's been helpful. That's what Mom would want for me, and it's how I can best honor her memory.

When you're ready, create a quiet, comfortable space where you can be undisturbed for a while, and explore the practice for yourself.

✏️ EXERCISE. Writing from My Multiple Selves

Situation:

Choose the emotion that is most prominent (anxious self/sad self/angry self). From the perspective of the emotional self you have chosen, write about the problem. Write about the external situation as well as your inner experiences (emotions, imagery, thoughts, bodily reactions, motives, etc.).

Chosen self:

Now write from another emotional self (anxious/sad/angry).

Chosen self:

Now write from another emotional self (anxious/sad/angry).

Chosen self:

Spend as long as you need to access and embody your compassionate self. When you are ready, write from the perspective of your compassionate self, addressing each emotional self as well as the external situation. From this compassionate perspective, how would you understand the perspectives of these emotional selves in relation to this difficult situation? How might you offer understanding, support, and encouragement to each of these emotional selves? How might this kind, wise, courageous, compassionate version of you work with this challenging situation?

Although space prevents us from demonstrating it, this is another practice that it can be useful to do as a limited co-therapy dyad, with the "therapist" providing prompts to the individual doing the exercise to shift into and explore the different emotional perspectives, and then facilitating the ability of the compassionate self to bring compassion to the various emotional selves and to the situation itself (an example of what such a dialogue might look like is included in Kolts, 2016, pp. 183–191).

Self-Reflective Questions

What was your experience of this multiple-selves writing exercise? How was it engaging in free-flowing writing? Did the process of writing down your thoughts and experiences add to the connection with each emotion? What are the clinical implications of this?

_____

_____

_____

_____

_____

_____

_____

_____

_____

_____

_____

_____

_____

_____

Did you notice any strong or difficult reactions to a particular emotional self? Did you notice any avoidance? Did you notice a preference for any particular emotional self? What do those reactions mean to you?

_____

_____

_____

_____

_____

_____

_____

_____

_____

_____

_____

_____

What was it like to bring compassion to different parts of yourself? Did you notice any blocks or difficulties? If so, how did you work with them?

_____

_____

_____

_____

_____

_____

_____

_____

_____

_____

_____

_____

_____

As a therapist, how might the presence of different emotional selves influence your therapy or supervision? Can you think of a client for whom such an exploration might be useful? How so?

_____

_____

_____

_____

_____

_____

_____

_____

_____

_____

_____

_____

How does your experience of the multiple selves practice relate to your understanding of the CFT model?

_____

_____

_____

_____

_____

_____

_____

_____

_____

_____

_____

_____

_____

MODULE 31

Attachment and the Professional Self

Throughout the book, we've focused on using SP/SR to help you learn CFT from the inside out. In doing so, you've brought your attention (and hopefully some compassion) to aspects of both your personal and professional lives. Many of the practices have likely oriented you to explore and bring compassion to issues arising in your personal life, and then we've tried to use bridging questions in the reflections to prompt consideration of how you might draw upon this personal experience in your professional work with clients, and in your understanding of CFT more broadly. As we're nearing the end of the book, we'll use the final few modules to focus more specifically on your professional self, and how we can bring compassionate exploration to understand and develop ourselves as therapists.

Module 10 focused on exploring attachment dynamics in your personal life. In this module, we'll use the lens of attachment to consider relationship dynamics in your professional life. Let's start by having you revisit the brief attachment questionnaire you've now seen several times. However, you may *notice that this version of the questionnaire has been altered so that the questions refer specifically to professional relationships*—your relationships with clients, colleagues, supervisors, supervisees, and the like. When answering, focus on one set of these relationships (e.g., clients or colleagues) at a time. Use your professional judgment as to the appropriateness of different types of interactions, and interpret the questions as referring to relationship-appropriate information (e.g., discussing therapy-relevant problems and concerns with a client would be appropriate, whereas it wouldn't be appropriate to explore workplace problems with clients—but such conversation would be appropriate to discuss with supervisors or colleagues). Also, you'll likely recall that the direction of the numbers changes in the middle of the measure due to the first four items being reverse-scored, so that all you need to do upon finishing is to sum up the scores that you've circled.

ECR-RS

Please read each of the following statements and rate the extent to which you believe each statement best describes your feelings about **your professional relationships.**	Strongly disagree						Strongly agree
1. It helps to turn to people in times of need.	7	6	5	4	3	2	1
2. I usually discuss my problems and concerns with others.	7	6	5	4	3	2	1
3. I usually talk things over with people.	7	6	5	4	3	2	1
4. I find it easy to depend on others.	7	6	5	4	3	2	1
5. I don't feel comfortable opening up to others.	1	2	3	4	5	6	7
6. I prefer not to show others how I feel deep down.	1	2	3	4	5	6	7
7. I often worry that others do not really care about me.	1	2	3	4	5	6	7
8. I'm afraid that other people may abandon me.	1	2	3	4	5	6	7
9. I worry that others won't care about me as much as I care about them.	1	2	3	4	5	6	7

Attachment Avoidance (sum items 1–6): _____

Attachment Anxiety (sum items 7–9): _____

As we've explored, a theme in CFT is that our life experiences shape us in ways we don't get to choose or design, but which profoundly influence our functioning in various life domains—and in the professional life of a therapist, it's perhaps difficult to find a more relevant example than our attachment patterns. Although many workplaces involve interacting with other people, our ability to form and maintain supportive relationships with others is particularly relevant to the professional life of therapists, as evidence suggests that the quality of the therapeutic relationship represents a primary determinant of client outcomes (Martin, Garske, & Davis, 2000). And while there's less definitive research speaking to the direct impact of therapist relationships with their colleagues and supervisors, it's safe to say that these relationships can have significant implications for the course of our professional lives. Starting with the now-familiar questions about attachment anxiety and avoidance you completed earlier in this module, the rest of the module guides you in reflecting upon your attachment experiences and how they influence various relationships in your professional life with clients, colleagues, and supervisors. Let's start by considering Joe's example.

EXAMPLE: Joe's Professional Attachments

In your current professional position, how do you experience your relationships? Do you feel comfortable forming relationships with clients, colleagues, and supervisors?

That's a tricky question. Previously in my career, I would have said that was no problem—up until my current position, I've always felt good about my relationships with people in the workplace—clients, colleagues, and supervisors. Of course, there were people who were harder to get to know, but that's to be expected. The dynamic at my new job is different, and it's definitely had me on edge—particularly with my supervisor, but also somewhat with colleagues, and to some extent with clients as well.

What are your relationships like with clients? Do you find it easy or challenging to form relationships with clients? Have any obstacles arisen in your relationships with clients?

I've generally been good at forming relationships with clients, and that's still mostly the case. My clients are the same as they've always been, coming to me for help. So although the relationships with my clients can be challenging sometimes, that doesn't really bother me, as it's easy to accept that working with those relationships is part of the work of therapy. In the new job, I've sometimes struggled staying as focused as I like in therapy if I've had frustrating interactions with my supervisor right beforehand, but I've started taking a few minutes before sessions to do some breathing and center my mind on the client who's coming in, and that's seemed to help.

What are your relationships like with colleagues? Do you have colleagues with whom you feel safe exploring problems and difficulties? Is it easy or difficult for you to feel close to your colleagues?

Things with colleagues are getting better. For a while, there seemed to be a competitive dynamic among all of us. There was such a focus on productivity that the stress level at work seemed to have people not trusting or connecting with one another, and for a while it was like parallel play—we'd all just put our heads down, see our clients, and go home without really interacting much—not even during staff meetings, where Gary (my supervisor) just tends to dominate things. I didn't like that, because it was really uncomfortable, and we need to be able to consult with one another about cases. It's just a lot nicer when people are getting along, like they did at the last place I worked. Luckily, we all went out for drinks about a month ago and got talking about Gary and how frustrating the situation was to all of us. We really seemed to bond over this sort of shared trauma we were experiencing at work. That helped, and things seem a lot better now. I've consulted with a couple of my colleagues about cases, and things feel a lot more comfortable. I've even gone running with one of them, who may end up becoming a close friend.

What are your relationships like with supervisors? Do you have supervisors with whom you feel safe exploring problems and difficulties? Is it easy or difficult for you to feel close to your supervisors?

This one is still a struggle. Historically, I've gotten along well with my supervisors and have felt pretty close to them, or at least felt like they had my back. Gary's not like that at all, but given what I've heard from my colleagues, that's about him, not me.

He still harps on and on about productivity, but all our numbers are in the acceptable range, so we've kind of learned to ignore him and focus on the job. Working through this program has helped me stop clinging to my anger at him and to put more energy into relationships that are helpful, like with my colleagues and family. That has helped a lot. I'm sort of hoping that Gary will end up taking another position somewhere—if that happened, I think I could have a good relationship with a new supervisor.

Given what you've described in your preceding answers, how might you bring compassion to your understanding of your professional relationships? Considering these relationships and your historical attachment dynamics, what would your compassionate self—the kindest, wisest, most courageous version of you—want you to understand about these relationships? How might this compassionate self validate, support, and encourage you as you take on the challenging relationships in your professional life?

A couple of things come to mind. First, my compassionate self would remind me that there are a lot of things about my job—most particularly, my supervisor and his behavior—that are out of my control, aren't my fault, and which are unlikely to change. Given that, it probably makes more sense for me to focus on accepting those things and working with the things I can affect to make the job as rewarding as it can be. I've been doing this more lately. I've been stewing a lot less about things (the breathing and imagery exercises have helped with that). It helps to remind myself that it isn't about me, that other people are struggling with the same things. Related to that, I feel good about finally having some satisfying relationships with my colleagues at work, and I want to put more into those connections. But I've been doing better with it—even my wife has noticed—so I guess my compassionate self would remind me of that and encourage me to keep going.

Can you identify any areas you'd like to grow or improve upon when it comes to working compassionately with this situation? What might be a step you could take in that direction?

Mostly, I want to maintain the progress I've made and build on it. I think I'll ask Alison [coworker] if she'd like to run together more regularly. Also, at my previous job we had a journal club for a while—it was a nice way to keep up with the literature a bit and have fun connections with my colleagues. It might be nice to have a journal club or book club. That would help me feel like I was doing something else to be at my best for my clients as well. On that note, I've also thought about seeking outside supervision once or twice a month. Gary's not helpful in that regard, but that doesn't mean I can't find a way to receive meaningful supervision.

Having considered Joe's experience, perhaps take a few minutes to get settled in, take a moment to review your responses on the ECR questionnaire, and then reflect upon your own experiences of attachment in your professional life.

EXERCISE. Exploring My Professional Attachments

In your current professional position, how do you experience your relationships? Do you feel comfortable forming relationships with clients, colleagues, and supervisors?

What are your relationships like with clients? Do you find it easy or challenging to form relationships with clients? Have any obstacles arisen in your relationships with clients?

What are your relationships with colleagues like? Do you have colleagues with whom you feel safe exploring problems and difficulties? Is it easy or difficult for you to feel close to your colleagues?

What are your relationships with supervisors like? Do you have supervisors with whom you feel safe exploring problems and difficulties? Is it easy or difficult for you to feel close to your supervisors?

Given what you've described in your preceding answers, how might you bring compassion to your understanding of your professional relationships? Considering these relationships and your historical attachment dynamics, what would your compassionate self—the kindest, wisest, most courageous version of you—want you to understand about these relationships? How might this compassionate self validate, support, and encourage you as you take on the challenging relationships in your professional life?

Can you identify any areas you'd like to grow or improve upon when it comes to working compassionately with this situation? What might be a step you could take in that direction?

Self-Reflective Questions

How was it focusing on the way in which your attachment style plays out in your professional life? What thoughts and feelings went through your mind as you considered these questions? Which motivational systems were aroused?

_____
_____
_____
_____
_____
_____
_____
_____
_____
_____

If any obstacles arose as you did the exercises, how did you work with them?

_____
_____
_____
_____
_____
_____
_____
_____
_____

_____

_____

_____

How does your experience of the attachment relationships in your professional life match with those in your personal life? What sense do you make of this?

_____

_____

_____

_____

_____

_____

_____

_____

_____

_____

_____

_____

How easy or difficult was it to feel compassion for yourself in the professional context? How does how you feel now compare with how you may have felt earlier in the SP/SR program? Are there any implications for your work with your clients?

_____

_____

_____

_____

_____

_____

_____

_____

_____

_____

_____

_____

How does your experience of this module affect your understanding of attachment theory?

_____

_____

_____

_____

_____

_____

_____

_____

_____

_____

_____

_____

_____

_____

MODULE 32

The Internal Compassionate Supervisor

As we've mentioned previously, it's useful to anchor therapy to process-level targets (e.g., increasing mindful awareness, cultivating compassionate motivation, building distress tolerance) rather than anchoring it to specific techniques. Based on the observation that many of the therapists they encountered identified feeling comfortable when extending compassion *to* others but often struggled to receive and make use of compassion offered *from* others, Bell, Dixon, and Kolts (2016) developed the internal compassionate supervisor exercise to target the other-to-self flow of compassion in a way that would specifically relate to therapists. This exercise is an adaptation of the "perfect nurturer" exercise developed by psychologist Deborah Lee (2005; itself an adaptation of Paul Gilbert's compassionate image practice), in which the client imagines being nurtured by an ideal compassionate being who is accepting, understanding, and helpful. This visualization exercise is similar to practices used in a number of spiritual traditions in which a spiritual being is focused on and connected with via prayer (e.g., Leighton, 2003). In CFT, we understand that our evolutionary heritage has shaped our brains to respond positively when we are cared for and supported by other people. The perfect nurturer practice uses mental imagery to access and harness the experience of being cared for, unconditionally, as a means to help us feel safe, supported, and soothed.

The term *internal supervisor* was first used by Patrick Casement (1985) to describe the way in which a supervisee forms an internalized representation of his or her supervisor and the supervision process (i.e., how the supervisor's ideas and viewpoints are integrated into the supervisee's own). In this exercise, we focus on using imagery to create a *compassionate* supervisor. Your internal compassionate supervisor will be an ideal fit for you, embodying and expressing compassionate qualities to support you in your clinical work as a therapist. These qualities might include strength and distress tolerance to help you face, tolerate, and work with the issues you might prefer to avoid in therapy, or you might choose a sense of warmth and kindness to help you feel safe and encouraged. Your internal supervisor might embody qualities of wisdom, helping you adopt a compassionate perspective toward the difficulties you encounter as a caring professional. It's important to remember that your compassionate supervisor is your own creation and is therefore perfect for you—knowing just what you need and what would be helpful to you. During the exercise, it can be beneficial to focus on your internal supervisor's compassionate commitment and intention, imagining that this inner creation is solely motivated to be helpful, to understand you completely, and to never let you down or criticize you. If you do find your image becoming critical or unkind, lacking in authority, or adopting qualities that are not helpful to you, refocus your mind on trying to create the qualities that you *would* find helpful from your supervisor.

Before we start the imagery exercise, use the questions in the following box (adapted from Gilbert, 2010) to consider what would make your compassionate supervisor ideal for you.

MY INTERNAL COMPASSIONATE SUPERVISOR

How would you like your compassionate supervisor to look (e.g., physical appearance, facial expressions)?

How would you like your compassionate supervisor to sound (e.g., tone of voice)?

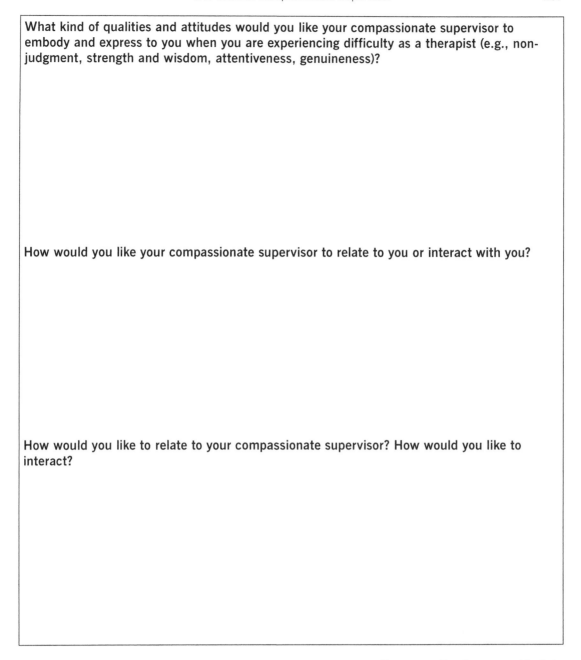

What kind of qualities and attitudes would you like your compassionate supervisor to embody and express to you when you are experiencing difficulty as a therapist (e.g., non-judgment, strength and wisdom, attentiveness, genuineness)?

How would you like your compassionate supervisor to relate to you or interact with you?

How would you like to relate to your compassionate supervisor? How would you like to interact?

Now, find a quiet place where you are unlikely to be disturbed. The exercise below takes around 15 minutes. Feel free to pause the exercise and do some soothing-rhythm breathing at any time, for as long as you may need, before bringing your attention back to the focus of the practice.

EXERCISE. Creating Your Internal Compassionate Supervisor

1. Begin by adopting a posture that is upright, open, comfortable, and alert. Close your eyes (or lower your gaze), relax your face, and allow your mouth to form a slight, warm, smile. Spend a minute practicing your soothing-rhythm breathing.

2. Bring to mind a comfortable, safe place where you would like to meet your compassionate supervisor.

3. When you feel soothed in your safe place, imagine your supervisor appearing before you. As you've noted previously, imagine your supervisor's physical appearance—his or her compassionate facial expression, posture, and movements. Imagine hearing his or her compassionate tone of voice (perhaps saying your name in a soothing way). Picture your supervisor sitting or standing beside you. Focus on how you might feel in the presence of this truly compassionate person, allowing yourself to be open to his or her kind attention and interest.

4. Imagine your supervisor embodying all the compassionate qualities that would be ideal for you and would help validate, support, and encourage your work as a therapist. Imagine how your supervisor would express and demonstrate these qualities to you and how you would feel receiving this compassion from them.

5. Now, let's focus on some specific qualities and attributes of your internal supervisor and how they relate to you in your role as a therapist:

   - *Wisdom.* Imagine that your compassionate supervisor has a deep wisdom, perhaps from his or her own personal experiences of pain and suffering, or his or her own development as a therapist over many years. Your supervisor truly understands the struggles you experience as a therapist, and will always help you to take a wise, compassionate perspective. This supervisor will see your experiences in a wider context, with the insight that, as humans, we are simply caught up in the flow of life, with a mind and emotions that are hard to manage. Imagine the empathy of your supervisor and your feeling of being deeply understood.

   - *Warmth.* Your supervisor also has great warmth, kindness, and unconditional caring for you. Imagine what it would be like to feel completely safe and accepted in the presence of your supervisor (don't worry if you do or don't feel safe and accepted; the key to the exercise is to imagine what it would be like *if you did*). Notice the feelings that would arise in you.

   - *Strength.* Imagine that your supervisor also embodies maturity, authority, and confidence. Your supervisor is not overwhelmed by your difficult experiences or your fears or frustrations, but remains present and responsive to whatever you bring. Imagine feeling your supervisor's confidence in you and in your ability to turn toward and work with the very things that you find difficult in therapy. Focus on the strength your supervisor gives you to be the best therapist you can be.

   - *Commitment.* Imagine that your supervisor is deeply committed to helping you work with your difficult experiences, and to providing you with the understanding, support, and encouragement to help you do so.

6. Imagine your supervisor speaking to you in a warm, supportive voice, conveying his or her care for, and commitment to, you in the form of the following wishes:

   - *"[Your name], may you be free of suffering."*
   - *"[Your name], may you be happy."*
   - *"[Your name], may you flourish."*
   - *"[Your name], may you find peace."*
   - Imagine hearing these wishes and hopes expressed to you for the following minute.

7. When you are ready, allow the image of your supervisor to fade. End the exercise by reconnecting with your soothing rhythm breathing. Open your eyes and readjust to the room.

After finishing the exercise, note your experiences below. In Joe's following example, he identifies his automatic, primary experiences (e.g., feeling anxious and his hands tensing up) and how he reacted and then related to those experiences (e.g., initially being critical but then switching his attention and using his body to reconnect with the exercise). You might want to reflect on both of these layers: automatic, primary experience (e.g., body sensations, emotions/feelings, initial thoughts or images) and then your response to such experiences.

 EXAMPLE: Joe's Reflection on the Internal Compassionate Supervisor Practice

What was your experience? What did you imagine? What did you notice in your body and emotions? How did you react or relate to your experiences?
*I thought this exercise would be very difficult, as I don't find my current supervisor that supportive. The word **supervisor** was a bit jarring at first because of that association. But during the exercise I started to think about what I need from a supervisor—what I need to feel safe enough to bring up the things I find difficult in doing therapy. My old supervisor flashed up, but then the image became someone else who had a lot of his qualities. Not being judged was key. I started to feel like anything that I said, thought, or felt would be okay and would be understood. I felt free. Then hearing those wishes felt strange—a bit intense when the image actually said my name. I noticed my body contracting and my hands tensing, and I felt anxious. I started to be a bit critical with myself, but I practiced returning my attention, opening my shoulders and hands, and lifting my head. It's something I want to go back to.*

 EXERCISE. My Reflection on the Internal Compassionate Supervisor Practice

What was your experience? What did you imagine? What did you notice in your body and emotions? How did you react or relate to your experiences?

Self-Reflective Questions

In what contexts can you imagine using your internal compassionate supervisor in the future?

_____

_____

_____

_____

_____

_____

_____

_____

Is there anything you might do differently in these different contexts?

_____

_____

_____

_____

_____

_____

_____

_____

_____

_____

Using Your Internal Compassionate Supervisor to Work with a Difficulty

In the previous module, you became acquainted with the internal compassionate supervisor practice. Now, we'll focus on putting your internal supervisor to work. Before trying this exercise, it is worth repeating the "Creation" exercise from Module 32 as many times as needed to get a good sense of your compassionate supervisor. As in all CFT imagery exercises, the aim is not to create an image with photographic clarity, but rather to create a *mental experience*—focusing on the felt sense that the image generates and your intention and willingness to develop these experiences of compassion.

In this exercise, you'll bring to mind a difficulty you've experienced as a therapist. This difficulty might be a working with a specific client, applying a particular intervention in therapy, or something more general about your role as a therapist. If you are practicing the exercise for the first time, choose a difficulty that doesn't cause you high levels of distress or discomfort.

EXERCISE. The Internal Compassionate Supervisor: Working with Difficulty

1. As with the previous exercise, close your eyes and begin your soothing rhythm breathing. Adopt a friendly facial expression and an open, comfortable, and alert posture.

   Bring to mind the image of your compassionate supervisor. Spend as long as you need imagining how he or she looks, sounds, moves, and interacts with you in a setting of your choice.

2. Now bring to mind a particular difficulty you're experiencing in your work as a therapist. This might be your work with a particular client, or an experience of therapy in which you feel somewhat stuck or reactive.

Imagine sharing your difficulty with your supervisor: sharing the nature of the problem and the details of what occurred, as well as your internal experiences (your thoughts, feelings, and impulses). You might notice a mixture of different emotions about the situation, such as anxiety, anger, hurt, or disappointment. See if you can allow and share them all.

You might imagine your supervisor helping you by gently asking the following questions:

- *What is it that you find upsetting or threatening about the situation?*
- *What is it that you fear?*
- *What part of you feels most vulnerable?*
- *What do you think this difficulty says about you and your abilities as a therapist?*
- *What part of you or your experience needs acceptance?*

Imagine sharing the very things you find difficult or frightening about this particular problem or scenario. Allow yourself to feel listened to by your supervisor with deep sensitivity, acceptance, and encouragement. Imagine feeling that you can tell your supervisor any aspect of your experience—your fantasies, fears, desires, and frustrations—and that your internal supervisor listens to everything with support and without judgment.

3. Next, imagine your compassionate supervisor showing you *kindness, care,* and *warmth* with regard to the difficulties you are experiencing. How would you like your supervisor to express this care? Hold in mind the supervisor's compassionate motivation: to be there solely to support you and your work. Imagine your supervisor's warm tone of voice and facial expression as he or she speaks to you and expresses words of genuine care and support. Notice how it would feel to receive this kindness and care. If you have difficulty accepting this care and kindness, imagine what it would be like *if you could accept it.* You might also imagine your supervisor bringing a sense of warmth and acceptance to any part of you that feels resistant to such care.

4. Now imagine your supervisor demonstrating a *deep understanding* of your experiences. Your supervisor understands that pain and difficulties are part of being human: part of having a tricky brain, of having nature's emotions and motivations flowing through you; part of being a caring professional and engaging with the suffering of others; and part of our conditioning as individuals. Your supervisor understands the challenges that can arise in therapy and the emotions that these challenges can trigger in us, and has a deep respect for the fact that you chose a career in which you would come directly into contact with peoples' suffering in order to help them. Imagine your supervisor expressing his or her empathy for you, understanding the reactions of your threat system and the ways in which these reactions can become intertwined with those of your clients or colleagues. Imagine how your supervisor might view your difficulties from a deeply compassionate perspective.

5. Next, focus on the *strength, authority,* and *maturity* your supervisor embodies and shares with you. Imagine your compassionate supervisor helping you to tolerate and approach the very things that are causing your distress, meeting these difficulties together with a sense of stability and strength. You might imagine that being with your supervisor gives you the maturity and confidence to accept and listen even more closely to the truth of your experience, your hurt, or your vulnerability, giving you the strength and confidence to learn from this struggle. Imagine having the personal authority to acknowledge areas of your practice that you want to improve. Your supervisor has faith in your abilities and resilience, and can see you growing from this experience.

6. Now, with a sense of warmth, understanding, and strength, imagine reflecting with your supervisor on *what you need.* Perhaps imagine speaking from the personal fears or vulnerabilities

you've identified: What do these fears or threats need to find peace or acceptance? What do you need to feel cared for and safe? What emotions or experiences might require caring attention? Imagine your supervisor offering you the care you need, and allow yourself to experience this care as fully as you can. If you do find any resistance in your emotions or thoughts, what might this part of you need to feel safe? What compassionate message might you need to hear to feel accepted and supported? Imagine your compassionate supervisor saying this message to you.

7. Finally, imagine discussing with your supervisor the most *skillful action* you could take. Your supervisor has a deep respect for your commitment to help others and is solely motivated to help you to become the therapist you want to be. Imagine reflecting with your supervisor on what action you could take to support both yourself and your clients in therapy, or to support your continuing development as a therapist. This action might involve a focus on how you can work compassionately with these difficulties the next time they occur. You might reflect on how to address these difficulties with your client. This action might also involve self-care for you personally, learning to support yourself in creating experiences of safeness and connection outside of the therapy room. Spend the next 30 seconds reflecting on potential actions you could take in your compassionate development as a therapist.

8. End the exercise by reconnecting with your soothing rhythm breathing and returning to your supervisor's unconditional wishes for you:

   - *May you be free of suffering.*
   - *May you be happy.*
   - *May you flourish.*
   - *May you find peace.*

   Give yourself as much time as you need to rest with your soothing rhythm breathing. When you are ready, allow the image of your supervisor to fade. Open your eyes and readjust yourself to your environment.

Once you have practiced the preceding exercise, take a look at Fatima's completed Compassionate Supervisor Worksheet (on page 304) to see how she engaged with the exercise. Then use the Compassionate Supervisor Worksheet on page 305 to document and further explore the perspective and support of your internal compassionate supervisor. Previous participants in a related research program (Bell et al., 2016) reported the most benefit when alternatively practicing the "Creation" and "Working with Difficulty" exercises from this module and Module 32 each day for 2 weeks. After 2 weeks, participants were able to access their inner supervisor quickly and independently, thereby integrating the exercise into their workday (e.g., using the worksheets after or before seeing a client whom they found difficult). Therefore, we suggest that you practice one of the internal supervisor exercises each day for the first 2 weeks, and then use the exercises as they suit you. If you choose to do this, we'd recommend that after the first few days of practicing the imagery exercises, you complete one of the following Compassionate Supervisor Worksheets every day (for 2 weeks) either before or after your clinical work.

FATIMA'S COMPASSIONATE SUPERVISOR WORKSHEET

	Your threat reaction, related fears, and self-critical thoughts	Bring to mind your inner compassionate supervisor and allow yourself to feel his or her support, care, and compassionate motivation. Imagine your supervisor sharing his or her compassionate perspective and wisdom, helping you understand your experiences and reactions from a position of safeness and strength. Use your compassionate supervisor to reframe your critical thoughts and help you focus on your potential to develop—to be the best therapist you can be. Imagine your supervisor taking in all aspects of your practice, widening your attention to take in positive elements and possibilities.
Situation or difficulty		
Working with a client with generalized anxiety disorder [GAD] and getting lost in all the worries.	I haven't taken this client to supervision because I'm embarrassed that I'm so many sessions in and still haven't figured out how to help her.	I'm sorry to hear that things have been difficult with your client. Given how busy you've been, both in and out of work, it makes sense that your resources feel low right now, doesn't it?
		It makes sense that your mind has been drawn to the things you feel are going wrong. Remember that this is your threat protection system working to help you by monitoring the things that threaten you as a therapist, such as how you might compare to other therapists. You care about your client and her well-being, and I'm pleased that you're concerned about her care and progress—it's a testament to your compassion and commitment. There are lots of things that you are doing well, both with this client and many others, but when you are feeling anxious and under threat, these things can naturally be difficult to remember. You've engaged this client well, and she has started to make changes.
	I don't like working with GAD. I should have done more reading and should have been more prepared. I felt anxious about interrupting her in the session—it felt rude and then too late, and I just switched off.	You've been able to identify areas you'd like to change in your work with this client. Acknowledging this, and how it makes you feel, is the beginning of compassion—you're showing real strength and honesty in doing this. You've felt uncertain before with other clients, and have learned and grown from these experiences. What are some first steps you could take to build your confidence in this area? You have wondered if your feelings of being overwhelmed and "switching off" are similar to how your client might be feeling—you can use this insight in your work. You could also speak to a colleague about the difficulties you are experiencing. Although it's difficult to do this when you're feeling insecure about how treatment is progressing, your colleagues will understand; they have all had similar experiences as therapists. In fact, you've helped them with exactly this sort of situation in the past, haven't you?
	I keep thinking she would be better off with another therapist.	Working with people in distress can be upsetting and stressful. You care so much about your work and the people you support. You need support too. It might be helpful to think about what you need too—in the next minutes, days, and week.
	I worry I'm not coping well.	I have every faith in your ability to continue growing and developing as a therapist. There is nothing wrong with you.

MY COMPASSIONATE SUPERVISOR WORKSHEET

Situation or difficulty	Your threat reaction, related fears, and self-critical thoughts	Bring to mind your inner compassionate supervisor and allow yourself to feel his or her support, care, and compassionate motivation. Imagine your supervisor sharing his or her compassionate perspective and wisdom, helping you understand your experiences and reactions from a position of safeness and strength. Use your compassionate supervisor to reframe your critical thoughts and help you focus on your potential to develop—to be the best therapist you can be. Imagine your supervisor taking in all aspects of your practice, widening your attention to take in positive elements and possibilities.

From *Experiencing Compassion-Focused Therapy from the Inside Out: A Self-Practice/Self-Reflection Workbook for Therapists* by Russell L. Kolts, Tobyn Bell, James Bennett-Levy, and Chris Irons. Published 2018 by The Guilford Press. Permission to photocopy this form is granted to purchasers of this book for personal use only (see copyright page for details). Purchasers can download additional copies of this form (see the box at the end of the table of contents).

Self-Reflective Questions

How did you experience developing and using your internal compassionate supervisor? Were there any surprises? Did you experience any difficulties?

_____

_____

_____

_____

_____

_____

_____

_____

_____

_____

_____

From your experience of developing and using your internal compassionate supervisor, can you identify any key threats, fears, or insecurities you frequently experience as a therapist? Have the exercises made you more aware of these?

_____

_____

_____

_____

_____

_____

_____

_____

_____

_____

_____

_____

How might you use your internal compassionate supervisor to support you during, before, or after therapy sessions?

_____

_____

_____

_____

_____

_____

_____

_____

_____

_____

_____

_____

From your experience of the exercises, how might you help clients or supervisees to develop their own "perfect nurturers" or ideal compassionate images? How will you help them work with difficulties they encounter when creating or using the imagery practices?

_____

_____

_____

_____

_____

_____

_____

_____

_____

_____

_____

_____

A number of the exercises in recent module have used mental imagery. How did you experience this? From this experience, what do you think is the value of using mental imagery in developing compassion? How does it relate to your understanding of CFT?

_____

_____

_____

_____

_____

_____

_____

_____

_____

_____

_____

_____

PART V

Reflecting on
Your CFT SP/SR Journey

MODULE 34

Maintaining and Enhancing Compassionate Growth

A primary goal in CFT involves empowering clients to develop compassionate strengths to help them work with both their presenting problems and with all they will face in their lives going forward. As we've discussed, CFT isn't really about teaching compassion techniques, but about helping clients cultivate *compassionate lives*—ways of being in the world characterized by kind curiosity, mindful awareness, compassionate wisdom, and the courageous willingness to engage and work with their experience, even when it is challenging and uncomfortable. *Especially* when it is challenging and uncomfortable.

As a course of therapy comes to an end, it is useful to reflect upon the journey with the client, and to create a plan for working compassionately with potential obstacles and challenges that may arise in the future, so we can set them up to continue the process of compassionate growth even when the therapy has ended. In this final module, we'll mirror that process by having you revisit the measures you've been using to track progress, reflect on the challenging problem you identified, and consider how you might build on growth you've observed during the program.

A second purpose of this final module involves reflecting upon your experience of SP/SR in relation to your professional development in CFT. You chose to engage in CFT "from the inside out" for various reasons, perhaps both professional and personal. What have you noticed about your experience? Have aspects of the experience been valuable to you? How might this process inform you professional and/or personal life going forward? Our hope is that you can take away things from your SP/SR experience with CFT that will contribute to both your continued professional development and to your personal life as a human being who, like everyone else, wants to be happy and to not suffer.

✐ **EXERCISE.** Revisiting the Measures

In the same manner as you've done before, rerate yourself on the measures below, just as you'd ask a client to do at the end of therapy.

ECR-RS: POST-SP/SR

Please read each of the following statements and rate the extent to which you believe each statement best describes your feelings about **close relationships in general.**	Strongly disagree						Strongly agree
1. It helps to turn to people in times of need.	7	6	5	4	3	2	1
2. I usually discuss my problems and concerns with others.	7	6	5	4	3	2	1
3. I usually talk things over with people.	7	6	5	4	3	2	1
4. I find it easy to depend on others.	7	6	5	4	3	2	1
5. I don't feel comfortable opening up to others.	1	2	3	4	5	6	7
6. I prefer not to show others how I feel deep down.	1	2	3	4	5	6	7
7. I often worry that others do not really care about me.	1	2	3	4	5	6	7
8. I'm afraid that other people may abandon me.	1	2	3	4	5	6	7
9. I worry that others won't care about me as much as I care about them.	1	2	3	4	5	6	7

Attachment Avoidance (sum items 1–6): _____

Attachment Anxiety (sum items 7–9): _____

FOCS ITEMS: POST-SP/SR

Please use this scale to rate the extent to which you agree with each statement.	Do not agree at all		Somewhat Agree		Completely Agree
1. Being too compassionate makes people soft and easy to take advantage of.	0	1	2	3	4
2. I fear that being too compassionate makes people an easy target.	0	1	2	3	4
3. I fear that if I am compassionate, some people will become dependent upon me.	0	1	2	3	4
4. I find myself holding back from feeling and expressing compassion toward others.	0	1	2	3	4
5. I try to keep my distance from others even if I know they are kind.	0	1	2	3	4
6. Feelings of kindness from others are somehow frightening.	0	1	2	3	4
7. When people are kind and compassionate toward me, I "put up a barrier."	0	1	2	3	4
8. I have a hard time accepting kindness and caring from others.	0	1	2	3	4
9. I worry that if I start to develop compassion for myself, I will become dependent upon it.	0	1	2	3	4
10. I fear that if I become too compassionate toward myself, I will lose my self-criticism and my flaws will show.	0	1	2	3	4
11. I fear that if I am more self-compassionate, I will become a weak person or my standards will drop.	0	1	2	3	4
12. I struggle with relating kindly and compassionately toward myself.	0	1	2	3	4

Note. This adaptation involves a limited selection of items from the FOC scale as well as additional summary items developed for this book. It was developed so that readers of this book could have a brief way of tracking their progress in working through the modules. As such, this selection of items has not been validated and is not appropriate for use in either research or clinical work. Readers can acquire a copy of the complete, validated version of the scale which is appropriate for research and clinical purposes at *https://compassionatemind.co.uk/resources/scales.*

Fears of Extending Compassion (sum items 1–4): _____
Fears of Receiving Compassion (sum items 5–8): _____
Fears of Self-Compassion (sum items 9–12): _____

Now for a final brief measure, the CEAS-SC.

CEAS-SC: POST-SP/SR

When I'm distressed or upset by things . . .	Never									Always
1. I am *motivated* to engage and work with my distress when it arises.	1	2	3	4	5	6	7	8	9	10
2. I *notice* and am *sensitive* to my distressed feelings when they arise in me.	1	2	3	4	5	6	7	8	9	10
3. I am *emotionally moved* by my distressed feelings or situations.	1	2	3	4	5	6	7	8	9	10
4. I *tolerate* the various feelings that are part of my distress.	1	2	3	4	5	6	7	8	9	10
5. I *reflect on* and *make sense* of my feelings of distress.	1	2	3	4	5	6	7	8	9	10
6. I am *accepting, noncritical,* and *non-judgmental* of my feelings of distress.	1	2	3	4	5	6	7	8	9	10
7. I direct my *attention* to what is likely to be helpful to me.	1	2	3	4	5	6	7	8	9	10
8. I *think* about and come up with helpful ways to cope with my distress.	1	2	3	4	5	6	7	8	9	10
9. I take the *actions* and do the things that will be helpful to me.	1	2	3	4	5	6	7	8	9	10
10. I create inner feelings of *support, helpfulness,* and *encouragement.*	1	2	3	4	5	6	7	8	9	10

> Compassionate Engagement (sum items 1–6): _____
>
> Compassionate Action (sum items 7–10):   _____

If you chose other measures that fit more specifically with your identified challenge or problem, you might want to complete them again as well. Now, reflecting upon your experience of the CFT SP/SR program, let's formally revisit your identified problem.

EXERCISE. Reflecting upon My Challenging Problem

My challenging problem:

What differences have you noticed in how you experience this challenging problem (or other challenges in your life)?

What compassion-based strategies or practices have you found most helpful as you have gone through the program? How so?

How will you support, develop, and strengthen your motivation and ability to engage with life compassionately in the future?

What internal (thoughts, emotions) or external (people, life challenges or crises) factors might get in the way of your compassionate ways of being?

What supports, resources, or practices might help you work with these blocks or obstacles?

Aside from this challenge or problem, what other effects from your participation in the CFT SP/SR program have you noticed in your personal life?

Now that you've reflected upon your experience of SP/SR in your personal life, let's consider what you've taken away from it in terms of your professional life.

 EXERCISE. Bringing Compassion to My Professional Life

How has engaging in this program from the inside out influenced your understanding of your clients' (or colleagues') experiences in working with their own problems and challenges?

Reflecting on your experience of the CFT SP/SR program, what have you learned that might be useful in your work with clients or in other aspects of your professional life?

Which strategies or practices from the program might be useful in your ongoing work with clients?

Conclusion

Thank you for choosing to join us in this journey of experiencing CFT from the inside out. We hope you've found the process helpful and informative. Compassion is based in the realization that life is hard, and that all of us will struggle and suffer sometimes. We're hopeful that you've found something in these pages that can help you meet the most challenging parts of your personal and professional life with kindness, courage, the willingness to accept and embrace all aspects of yourself, and the confidence that, whatever arises, *you can work with this, too.* We also hope that in exploring CFT in this way, you've taken away some experiences that will be helpful in your work with your clients. Finally, we'd like to offer one last practice suggestion: From the perspective of your kind, wise, and courageous compassionate self, honor the beautiful commitment you've made to helping others with their suffering—the commitment that brought you to this book and to your work. This courageous commitment is the core of compassion, and it is worth celebrating!

Self-Reflective Questions

How would you sum up your experience of *Experiencing CFT from the Inside Out?*

_____

_____

_____

_____

_____

_____

_____

_____

_____

_____

_____

_____

_____

In reflecting upon your experience of completing the program, what do you see as the most important "take-home" messages?

For your professional life:

_____

_____

_____

_____

_____

_____

_____

_____

_____

_____

_____

_____

_____

_____

For your personal life:

_____

_____

_____

_____

_____

_____

_____

_____

_____

_____

_____

_____

_____

Do you think it would be valuable to continue using an SP/SR approach in the future? How so? What might you do? What could you do to weave it into your professional life? What obstacles might get in the way, and how might you work with them?

_____

_____

_____

_____

_____

_____

_____

_____

_____

_____

_____

_____

_____

_____

References

Bandura, A. (1977). *Social learning theory.* Englewood Cliffs, NJ: Prentice Hall.

Bell, T., Dixon, A., & Kolts, R. (2016). Developing a compassionate internal supervisor: Compassion-focused therapy for trainee therapists. *Clinical Psychology and Psychotherapy, 24,* 632–648.

Bennett-Levy, J. (2006). Therapist skills: A cognitive model of their acquisition and refinement. *Behavioural and Cognitive Psychotherapy, 34,* 57–78.

Bennett-Levy, J., Butler, G., Fennell, M., Hackmann, A., Mueller, M., & Westbrook, D. (Eds.). (2004). *The Oxford guide to behavioural experiments in cognitive therapy.* Oxford, UK: Oxford University Press.

Bennett-Levy, J., & Finlay-Jones, A. (in press). The role of personal practice in therapist skill development: A model to guide therapists, educators, supervisors and researchers. *Cognitive Behavior Therapy.*

Bennett-Levy, J., & Haarhoff, B. (in press). Why therapists need to take a good look at themselves: Self-practice/self-reflection as an integrative training strategy for evidence-based practices. In S. Dimidjian (Ed.), *Evidence-based behavioral practice in action.* New York: Guilford Press.

Bennett-Levy, J., & Lee, N. (2014). Self-practice and self-reflection in cognitive behaviour therapy training: What factors influence trainees' engagement and experience of benefit? *Behavioural and Cognitive Psychotherapy, 42,* 48–64.

Bennett-Levy, J., Lee, N., Travers, K., Pohlman, S., & Hamernik, E. (2003). Cognitive therapy from the inside: Enhancing therapist skills through practising what we preach. *Behavioural and Cognitive Psychotherapy, 31,* 145–163.

Bennett-Levy, J., McManus, F., Westling, B., & Fennell, M. J. V. (2009). Acquiring and refining CBT skills and competencies: Which training methods are perceived to be most effective? *Behavioural and Cognitive Psychotherapy, 37,* 571–583.

Bennett-Levy, J., Thwaites, R., Chaddock, A., & Davis, M. (2009). Reflective practice in cognitive behavioural therapy: The engine of lifelong learning. In J. Stedmon & R. Dallos (Eds.), *Reflective practice in psychotherapy and counselling* (pp. 115–135). Maidenhead, UK: Open University Press.

Bennett-Levy, J., Thwaites, R., Haarhoff, B., & Perry, H. (2015). *Experiencing CBT from the Inside Out: A self-practice/self-reflection workbook for therapists.* New York: Guilford Press.

Bennett-Levy, J., Turner, F., Beaty, T., Smith, M., Paterson, B., & Farmer, S. (2001). The value of self-practice of cognitive therapy techniques and self-reflection in the training of cognitive therapists. *Behavioural and Cognitive Psychotherapy, 29,* 203–220.

Berntson, G. G., Cacioppo, J. T., & Quigley, K. S. (1993). Respiratory sinus arrhythmia: Autonomic origins, physiological mechanisms, and psychophysiological implications. *Psychophysiology, 30,* 183–196.

Berry, K., & Danquah, A. (2016). Attachment-informed therapy for adults: Towards a unifying perspective on practice. *Psychology and Psychotherapy, 89,* 15–32.

Black, S., Hardy, G., Turpin, G., & Parry, G. (2005). Self-reported attachment styles and therapeutic orientation of therapists and their relationship with reported general alliance quality and problems in therapy. *Psychology and Psychotherapy, 78,* 363–377.

Bolton, G. (2010). *Reflective practice: Writing and professional development* (3rd ed.). London: SAGE.

Bowlby, J. (1980). *Attachment and loss: Vol. 3. Loss, sadness and depression.* London: Hogarth Press.

Bowlby, J. (1982) *Attachment and loss: Vol.1. Attachment.* London: Hogarth Press and the Institute of Psycho-Analysis. (Original work published 1969)

Bowlby, J. (1988). *A secure base: Clinical applications of attachment theory.* London: Routledge.

Brown, R. P., & Gerbarg, P. L. (2005). Sudarshan Kriya yogic breathing in the treatment of stress, anxiety, and depression: Part I—neurophysiologic model. *Journal of Alternative and Complementary Medicine, 11,* 189–201.

Burns, D. D. (1980). *Feeling good: The new mood therapy.* New York: New American Library.

Cameron, K., Mora, C., Leutscher, T., & Calarco, M. (2011). Effects of positive practices on organizational effectiveness. *Journal of Applied Behavioral Science, 47,* 266–308.

Carter, R. (2008). *Multiplicity: The new science of personality.* London: Little Brown.

Casement, P. (1985). *On learning from the patient.* London: Tavistock.

Chaddock, A., Thwaites, R., Bennett-Levy, J., & Freeston, M. (2014). Understanding individual differences in response to self-practice and self-reflection (SP/SR) during CBT training. *The Cognitive Behaviour Therapist, 7,* e14.

Davis, M. L., Thwaites, R., Freeston, M. H., & Bennett-Levy, J. (2015). A measurable impact of a self-practice/self-reflection programme on the therapeutic skills of experienced cognitive-behavioural therapists. *Clinical Psychology and Psychotherapy, 22,* 176–184.

Desbordes, G., Negi, L. T., Pace, T. W., Wallace, B. A., Raison, C. L., & Schwartz, E. L. (2012). Effects of mindful-attention and compassion meditation training on amygdala response to emotional stimuli in an ordinary, non-meditative state. *Frontiers in Human Neuroscience, 6,* 292.

Farrand, P., Perry, J., & Linsley, S. (2010). Enhancing self-practice/self-reflection (SP/SR) approach to cognitive behaviour training through the use of reflective blogs. *Behavioural and Cognitive Psychotherapy, 38,* 473–477.

Feeney, B. C., & Thrush, R. L. (2010). Relationship influences upon exploration in adulthood: The characteristics and function of a secure base. *Journal of Personality and Social Psychology, 98,* 57–76.

Finlay-Jones, A. L., Rees, C. S., & Kane, R. T. (2015). Self-compassion, emotion regulation and stress among Australian psychologists: Testing an emotion regulation model of self-compassion using structural equation modeling. *PLOS ONE, 10*, e0133481.

Fraley, R. C., Hefferman, M. E., Vicary, A. M., & Brumbaugh, C. C. (2011). The Experiences in Close Relationships—Relationship Structures Questionnaire: A method for assessing attachment orientations across relationships. *Psychological Assessment, 23*, 612–625.

Frederickson, B. L., Cohn, M. A., Coffee, K. A., Pek, J., & Finkel, S. M. (2008). Open hearts build lives: Positive emotions, induced through loving-kindness meditation, build consequential personal resources. *Journal of Personality and Social Psychology, 95*, 1045–1062.

Gale, C., & Schröder, T. (2014). Experiences of self-practice/self-reflection in cognitive behavioural therapy: A meta-synthesis of qualitative studies. *Psychology and Psychotherapy: Theory, Research and Practice, 87*, 373–392.

Gale, C., Schröder, T., & Gilbert, P. (2017). "Do you practice what you preach?": A qualitative exploration of therapists' personal practice of compassion focused therapy. *Clinical Psychology and Psychotherapy, 24*, 171–185.

Germer, C. K., & Neff, K. (2013). Self-compassion in clinical practice. *Journal of Clinical Psychology: In Session, 69*, 856–867.

Germer, C. K., & Neff, K. (2017). *Mindful self-compassion teacher guide*. San Diego: Center for MSC.

Gilbert, P. (1984). *Depression: From psychology to brain state*. Mahwah, NJ: Erlbaum.

Gilbert, P. (2009). *The compassionate mind*. London: Constable & Robinson.

Gilbert, P. (2010). *Compassion-focused therapy: Distinctive features*. London: Routledge.

Gilbert, P. (2014). The origins and nature of compassion focused therapy. *British Journal of Clinical Psychology, 53*, 6–41.

Gilbert, P. (2015). The evolution and social dynamics of compassion. *Social and Personality Psychology Compass, 9*, 239–254.

Gilbert, P., Caterino, F., Duarte, C., Matos, M., Kolts, R., Stubbs, J., et al. (2017). The development of compassionate engagement and action scales for self and others. *Journal of Compassionate Health Care, 4*.

Gilbert, P., & Choden. (2013). *Mindful compassion*. London: Robinson.

Gilbert, P., & Irons, C. (2005). Focused therapies and compassionate mind training for shame and self-attacking. In P. Gilbert (Ed.), *Compassion: Conceptualisations, research and use in psychotherapy* (pp. 9–74). London: Routledge.

Gilbert, P., McEwan, K., Catarino, F., Baião, R., & Palmeira, L. (2014). Fears of happiness and compassion in relationship with depression, alexithymia, and attachment security in a depressed sample. *British Journal of Clinical Psychology, 53*, 228–244.

Gilbert, P., McEwan, K., Matos, M., & Rivis, A. (2011). Fears of compassion: Development of three self-report measures. *Psychology and Psychotherapy: Theory, Research and Practice, 84*, 239–255.

Gillath, O., Shaver, P. R., & Mikulincer, M. (2005). An attachment-theoretical approach to compassion and altruism. In P. Gilbert (Ed.), *Compassion: Conceptualisations, research, and use in psychotherapy* (pp. 121–147). London: Routledge.

Greenberg, L. S. (2002). *Emotion-focused therapy: Coaching clients to work through their feelings*. Washington, DC: American Psychological Association.

Greenberger, D., & Padesky, C. A. (2015). *Mind over mood* (2nd ed.). New York: Guilford Press.

Haarhoff, B. (2006). The importance of identifying and understanding therapist schema in cognitive therapy training and supervision. *New Zealand Journal of Psychology, 35,* 126–131.

Haarhoff, B., Gibson, K., & Flett, R. (2011). Improving the quality of cognitive behaviour therapy case conceptualization: The role of self-practice/self-reflection. *Behavioural and Cognitive Psychotherapy, 39,* 323–339.

Haarhoff, B., & Thwaites, R. (2016). *Reflection in CBT.* London: Sage.

Haarhoff, B., Thwaites, R., & Bennett-Levy, J. (2015). Engagement with self-practice/self-reflection as professional development: The role of therapist beliefs. *Australian Psychologist, 50,* 322–328.

Hanson, R., & Mendius, R. (2009). *Buddha's brain: The practical neuroscience of happiness, love and wisdom.* Oakland, CA: New Harbinger.

Hutcherson, C. A., Seppälä, E. M., & Gross, J. J. (2008). Loving-kindness meditation increases social connectedness. *Emotion, 8,* 720–724.

Hutcherson, C. A., Seppälä, E. M., & Gross, J. J. (2015). The neural correlates of social connection. *Cognitive, Affective, and Behavioral Neuroscience, 15,* 1–15.

Irons, C., & Beaumont, E. (2017). *The compassionate mind workbook.* London: Robinson.

Jazaieri, H., McGonigal, K., Jinpa, T., Doty, J. R., Gross, J. J., & Goldin, P. R. (2013). A randomized controlled trial of compassion cultivation training: Effects on mindfulness, affect, and emotion regulation. *Motivation and Emotion, 38,* 23–35.

Jerath, R., Edry, J. W., Barnes, V. A., & Jerath, V. (2006). Physiology of long pranayamic breathing: Neural respiratory elements may provide a mechanism that explains how slow deep breathing shifts the autonomic nervous system. *Medical Hypotheses, 67,* 566–571.

Kabat-Zinn, J. (2013). *Full catastrophe living: How to cope with stress, pain and illness using mindfulness meditation* (2nd ed.). London: Piatkus.

Kaeding, A., Sougleris, C., Reid, C., van Vreeswijk, M. F., Hayes, C., Dorrian, J., et al. (2017). Professional burnout, early maladaptive schemas, and physical health in clinical and counseling psychology trainees. *Journal of Clinical Psychology, 73,* 1782–1796.

Kaushik, R. M., Kaushik, R., Mahajan, S. K., & Rajesh, V. (2006). Effects of mental relaxation and slow breathing in essential hypertension. *Complementary Therapies in Medicine, 14,* 120–126.

Kemeny, M. E., Foltz, C., Cavanagh, J. F., Cullen, M., Giese-Davis, J., Jennings, P., et al. (2012). Contemplative/emotion training reduces negative emotional behavior and promotes prosocial responses. *Emotion, 12,* 338–350.

Knox, J. (2010). *Self-agency in psychotherapy: Attachment, autonomy, and intimacy.* New York: Norton.

Kok, B. E., & Frederickson, B. L. (2010). Upwards spirals of the heart: Autonomic flexibility, as indexed by vagal tone, reciprocally and prospectively predicts positive emotions and social connectedness. *Biological Psychology, 85,* 432–436.

Kolts, R. L. (2011). *The compassionate mind approach to managing your anger.* London: Robinson.

Kolts, R. L. (2016). *CFT made simple.* Oakland, CA: New Harbinger.

LeDoux, J. (1998). *The emotional brain.* London: Weidenfeld & Nicolson.

Lee, D. A. (2005). The perfect nurturer: A model to develop compassionate mind within the context of cognitive therapy. In P. Gilbert (Ed.), *Compassion: Conceptualisations, research and use in psychotherapy* (pp. 236–251). Hove, UK: Routledge.

Leiberg, S., Limecki, O., & Singer, T. (2011). Short-term compassion training increases prosocial behavior in a newly developed prosocial game. *PLOS ONE, 6*, e17798.

Leighton, T. (2003). *Faces of compassion: Classic Bodhisattva archetypes and their modern expression*. Boston: Wisdom.

Lutz, A., Brefczynski-Lewis, J., Johnstone, T., & Davidson, R. J. (2008). Regulation of the neural circuitry of emotion by compassion meditation: Effects of meditative expertise. *PLOS ONE*, e1897.

Martin, D. J., Garske, J. P., & Davis, K. M. (2000). Relation of the therapeutic alliance with outcome and other variables: A meta-analytic review. *Journal of Consulting and Clinical Psychology, 68*, 438–450.

Mascaro, J. S., Rilling, J. K., Negi, L. T., & Raison, C. I. (2013). Compassion meditation enhances empathic accuracy and related neural activity. *Social Cognitive and Affective Neuroscience, 8*, 48–55.

McMillan, D., & Lee, R. (2010). A systematic review of behavioral experiments vs. exposure alone in the treatment of anxiety disorders: A case of exposure while wearing the emperor's new clothes? *Clinical Psychology Review, 30*, 467–478.

Mikulincer, M., Gillath, O., Halevy, V., Avihou, N., Avidan, S., & Eshkoli, N. (2001). Attachment theory and reactions to others' needs: Evidence that activation of the sense of attachment security promotes empathic responses. *Journal of Personality and Social Psychology, 81*, 1205–1224.

Mikulincer, M., & Shaver, P. R. (2005). Attachment security, compassion, and altruism. *Current Directions in Psychological Science, 14*, 34–38.

Mikulincer, M., & Shaver, P. R. (2007). *Attachment in adulthood: Structure, dynamics, and change*. New York: Guilford Press.

Mikulincer, M., & Shaver, P. R. (2012). An attachment perspective on psychopathology. *World Psychiatry, 11*, 11–15.

Mikulincer, M., & Shaver, P. R. (2016). *Attachment in adulthood: Structure, dynamics, and change* (2nd ed.). New York: Guilford Press.

Mikulincer, M., Shaver, P. R., & Berant, E. (2013). An attachment perspective on therapeutic processes and outcomes. *Journal of Personality, 81*, 606–616.

Neff, K. (2011). *Self-compassion: The proven power of being kind to yourself*. New York: William Morrow.

Neff, K. D., Kirkpatrick, K., & Rude, S. S. (2007). Self-compassion and its link to adaptive psychological functioning. *Journal of Research in Personality, 41*, 139–154.

Neff, K. D., & McGehee, P. (2010). Self-compassion and psychological resilience among adolescents and young adults, *Self and Identity, 9*, 225–240.

Pace, T. W. W., Negi, L. T., Adame, D. D., Cole, S. P., Sivilli, T. I., Brown, T. D., et al. (2009). Effect of compassion meditation on neuroendocrine, innate immune and behavioral responses to psychological stress. *Psychoneuroendocrinology, 34*, 87–98.

Pace, T. W. W., Negi, L. T., Dodson-Lavelle, B., Ozawa-de Silva, B., Reddy, S. D., Cole, S. P., et al. (2013). Engagement with cognitively-based compassion training is associated with reduced salivary C-reactive protein from before to after training in foster care program adolescents. *Psychoneuroendocrinology, 38*, 294–299.

Pakenham, K. I. (2015). Effects of acceptance and commitment therapy (ACT) training on clinical psychology trainee stress, therapist skills and attributes, and ACT processes. *Clinical Psychology and Psychotherapy, 22,* 647–655.

Pal, G. K., & Velkumary, S. (2004). Effect of short-term practice of breathing exercises on autonomic functions in normal human volunteers. *Indian Journal of Medical Research, 120,* 115–121.

Panksepp, J., & Biven, L. (2012). *The archaeology of mind: Neuroevolutionary origins of human emotions.* New York: Norton.

Patsiopoulos, A. T., & Buchanan, M. J. (2011). The practice of self-compassion in counseling: A narrative inquiry. *Professional Psychology: Research and Practice, 42,* 301–307.

Pennebaker, J. W. (1997). Writing about emotional experiences as a therapeutic process. *Psychological Science, 8,* 162–166.

Pennebaker, J. W. (2004). *Writing to heal: A guided journal for recovering from trauma and emotional upheaval.* Oakland, CA: New Harbinger.

Pepping, C. A., Davis, P. J., O'Donovan, A., & Pal, J. (2014). Individual difference in self-compassion: The role of attachment and experiences of parenting in childhood. *Self and Identity, 14,* 104–117.

Porges, S. W., Doussard-Roosevelt, J. A., & Maiti, A. K. (1994). Vagal tone and the physiological regulation of emotion. *Monographs of the Society for Research in Child Development, 59,* 167–186.

Raab, K. (2014). Mindfulness, self-compassion, and empathy among health care professionals: A review of the literature. *Journal of Health Care Chaplaincy, 20,* 95–108.

Ramnerö, J., & Törneke, N. (2008). *The ABCs of human behavior: Behavioral principles for the practicing clinician.* Oakland, CA: New Harbinger.

Reese, R. J., Norsworthy, L. A., & Rowlands, S. R. (2009). Does a continuous feedback system improve psychotherapy outcome? *Psychotherapy: Theory, Research, Practice, and Training, 4,* 418–431.

Rogers, C. R. (1951). *Client-centred therapy.* Boston: Houghton Mifflin.

Rønnestad, M. H., & Skovholt, T. M. (2003). The journey of the counselor and therapist: Research findings and perspectives on professional development. *Journal of Career Development, 30,* 5–44.

Salkovskis, P. M., Hackmann, A., Wells, A., Gelder, M. G., & Clark, D. M. (2007). Belief disconfirmation versus habituation approaches to situational exposure in panic disorder with agoraphobia: A pilot study. *Behaviour Research and Therapy, 45,* 877–885.

Salzberg, S. (2002). *Lovingkindness: The revolutionary art or happiness.* Boston: Shambhala.

Sanders, D., & Bennett-Levy, J. (2010). When therapists have problems: What can CBT do for us? In M. Mueller, H. Kennerley, F. McManus, & D. Westbrook (Eds.), *The Oxford guide to surviving as a CBT therapist* (pp. 457–480). Oxford, UK: Oxford University Press.

Schön, D. A. (1983). *The reflective practitioner.* New York: Basic Books.

Segal, Z. V., Williams, J. M. G., & Teasdale, J. D. (2012). *Mindfulness-based cognitive therapy for depression.* New York: Guilford Press.

Seppälä, E. (2016). *The happiness track.* New York: HarperCollins.

Skinner, B. F. (1953). *Science and human behavior.* New York: Macmillan.

Spafford, S., & Haarhoff, B. (2015). What are the conditions needed to facilitate online self-reflection for CBT trainees? *Australian Psychologist, 50,* 232–240.

Spendelow, J. S., & Butler, L. J. (2016). Reported positive and negative outcomes associated with a self-practice/self-reflection cognitive-behavioural therapy exercise for CBT trainees. *Psychotherapy Research, 26,* 602–611.

Stott, R. (2007). When head and heart do not agree: A theoretical and clinical analysis of rational-emotional dissociation (RED) in cognitive therapy. *Journal of Cognitive Psychotherapy: An International Quarterly, 21,* 37–50.

Teasdale, J. D. (1996). Clinically relevant theory: Integrating clinical insight with cognitive science. In P. M. Salkovskis (Ed.), *Frontiers of cognitive therapy* (pp. 26–47). New York: Guilford Press.

Teasdale, J. D. (1999). Metacognition, mindfulness and the modification of mood disorders. *Clinical Psychology and Psychotherapy, 6,* 146–155.

Thwaites, R., Bennett-Levy, J., Cairns, L., Lowrie, R., Robinson, A., Haarhoff, B., et al. (2017). Self-practice/self-reflection (SP/SR) as a training strategy to enhance therapeutic empathy in low intensity CBT practitioners. *New Zealand Journal of Psychology, 46,* 63–70.

Thwaites, R., Bennett-Levy, J., Davis, M., & Chaddock, A. (2014). Using self-practice and self-reflection (SP/SR) to enhance CBT competence and meta-competence. In A. Whittington & N. Grey (Eds.), *How to become a more effective CBT therapist: Mastering metacompetence in clinical practice* (pp. 241–254). Chichester, UK: Wiley-Blackwell.

Thwaites, R., Cairns, L., Bennett-Levy, J., Johnston, L., Lowrie, R., Robinson, A., et al. (2015). Developing metacompetence in low intensity CBT interventions: Evaluating a self-practice/self-reflection program for experienced low intensity CBT practitioners. *Australian Psychologist, 50,* 311–321.

Villatte, M., Villatte, J. L., & Hayes, S. C. (2016). *Mastering the clinical conversation.* New York: Guilford Press.

Wallin, D. J. (2007). *Attachment in psychotherapy.* New York: Guilford Press.

Welford, M. (2016). *Compassion focused therapy for dummies.* Chichester, UK: Wiley.

Index

Note. *f* or *t* following a page number indicates a figure or a table.